Written Assessment in Medical Education

Hosam Eldeen Elsadig Gasmalla
Alaa AbuElgasim Mohamed Ibrahim
Majed M. Wadi • Mohamed H. Taha
Editors

# Written Assessment in Medical Education

Springer

*Editors*
Hosam Eldeen Elsadig Gasmalla
University of Warwick
Coventry, United Kingdom

Al-Neelain University
Khartoum, Sudan

Majed M. Wadi
Medical Education Department College of Medicine
Qassim University
Buraidah, Saudi Arabia

Alaa AbuElgasim Mohamed Ibrahim
College of Oral and Dental Medicine
Karary University
Khartoum, Sudan

Educational Development Center
Sudan Medical Spacialization Board
Khartoum, Sudan

Mohamed H. Taha
College of Medicine and Medical Education
Centre University of Sharjah
Sharjah, United Arab Emirates

ISBN 978-3-031-11754-1 ISBN 978-3-031-11752-7 (eBook)
https://doi.org/10.1007/978-3-031-11752-7



This Springer imprint is published by the registered company Springer Nature Switzerland AG
The registered company address is: Gewerbestrasse 11, 6330 Cham, Switzerland

# Preface

Assessment lies at the heart of any educational process. For education in medical and health professions, assessment is extremely important since the decision taken after assessment affects the lives of people. From this notion, assessment should be robust and credentialed. The assessment should be tailored to appraise the level of medical graduate competencies, who will offer healthcare to patients and serve the health system. It must clearly state and support the criteria for their certification.

Over the last four decades, health professions schools, postgraduate residency programs, and licensing agencies have all expanded their efforts to provide accurate, reliable, and timely assessments of students, trainees, and practicing physicians' competencies. The three major purposes of such assessments are to maximize the capacities of all learners and practitioners by giving incentives and guidance for future learning, to safeguard the public by detecting incompetent physicians, and to offer a framework for selecting advanced training applicants.

Despite the availability of many educational resources, faculty development programs, the emergence of new global challenges and the fourth industrial revolution, and the COVID-19 pandemic, which created a new normal, topics of assessment continue to be challenging for faculty, particularly novices. Therefore, the purpose of this book is to provide readers with an understanding of the fundamentals of written assessment and to provide a simple guide for daily use by a medical educator. We merely focused on written assessment since written assessment topics continue to be highly in demand by faculty members, who frequently request and participate in numerous training activities under this umbrella. This book does not overwhelm the reader with an abundance of educational theory; rather, it serves the needs of medical educators in a straightforward and uncomplicated manner.

In writing this book, we used a simplified description of the theory, followed by practical tips and examples from daily practice in health professions education schools, as well as practical exercises. Finally, each chapter ends with a take-home message. The book is organized into 14 chapters.

Chapter 1 introduces basic assessment concepts, highlighting the various types of assessment methods, as well as the criteria that define a good assessment. The second chapter sheds light on assessing learning outcomes using various theoretical foundations such as Miller's pyramid and Bloom's taxonomy. Chapter 3 provides a step-by-step guide for designing and developing a test blueprint. It also includes several examples of various blueprints. Chapter 4 goes over the various formats of constructed response items, their strengths and weaknesses, and how to construct them. Chapter 5 explains the concept of key-feature questions (KFQs), their structure, and evidence to support their validity. Chapter 6 focuses on the development of A-type MCQs that go beyond assessing recall to assessing high levels of the cognitive domain, with extensive use of examples. Chapter 7 explains R-type questions and describes their structure and how to construct high-quality R-Type MCQs. Chapter 8 aims at introducing readers to the Script Concordance Test and its psychometric properties, as well as its use in medical education. Chapter 9 aims to introduce readers to the statistical methods used in exam evaluation through simple and descriptive examples. Chapter 10 sheds light on the standard-setting process and discusses relevant methods used in written exams. The importance of online assessment as an emerging strategy for evaluating and monitoring students' achievement in e-learning is highlighted in Chap. 11. Chapter 12 introduces the readers to progress testing in written assessment, including the rationale for the test, how to run it, and how to evaluate it. Chapter 13 discusses the fundamental principles of programmatic assessment as well as the conceptual and theoretical frameworks that support it. Chapter 14 focuses on social accountability SA in the written assessment and how to integrate SA values into assessment practice.

We believe that the book will serve educators in medical and health professions in planning, designing, and implementing different assessment activities within their context.

We are especially grateful to all our authors, who took time out of their hectic professional schedules to make an outstanding contribution to book chapters.

Finally, we would like to thank our families for their patience with our numerous distractions during the lengthy timeline required to complete this book.

Coventry, United Kingdom — Hosam Eldeen Elsadig Gasmalla
Khartoum, Sudan — Alaa AbuElgasim Mohamed Ibrahim
Buraidah, Saudi Arabia — Majed M. Wadi
Sharjah, United Arab Emirates — Mohamed H. Taha

May 2022
hosam.mohammed@warwick.ac.uk
M.wadi@qu.edu.sa

# Contents

# Notes on the Editors

**Hosam Eldeen Elsadig Gasmalla, MBBS, MSc, PgDip, MHPE, PhD** is Assistant Professor of Clinical Anatomy and medical education specialist in the Faculty of Medicine, Al-Neelain University, Sudan, with over 15 years of experience in teaching and research in both clinical anatomy and medical/health professions education for undergraduates and graduate students. Dr. Hosam Eldeen is specialized in students' assessment, and he teaches learners' assessment module as part of the master's degree program in health professions education provided by the Sudan Medical Specialization Board (SMSB). Dr. Hosam Eldeen also has experience in the field of quality of education. As a founding dean, he established and led the deanship of quality and education development at Sudan International University (2020–2022). He is also a member of several international organizations including the Association for Medical Education in Europe (AMEE). Recently, he moved to the United Kingdom as an Assistant Professor of Clinical Anatomy at The University of Warwick.

**hosam.mohammed@warwick.ac.uk**

**Alaa Abuelgasim Mohamed Ibrahim, MDDPH, MHPE, MPTH** is the dean of the College of Oral and Dental Medicine at Karary University and Assistant Professor of Dental Public Health (DPH). Dr. Alaa also serves on the Sudan Medical Specialization Board (SMSB) as the head of the curriculum and program department at the Education Development Center, as the rapporteur of the curriculum high advice committee, and as the dental public health counsel rapporteur. She contributes to health professions education (HPE) by serving as the main instructor for the master's degree program in HPE at SMSB and the International University of Africa, facilitating HPE and DPH courses in Sudanese universities for more than 8 years, and designing undergraduate and postgraduate curricula for various health professional programs for more than 5 years.

**Majed Wadi, MBBS, MSc Med Edu** is a lecturer in the Medical Education Department of the College of Medicine, Qassim University, Saudi Arabia. Dr.

Majed has vast expertise with student assessment as he is the coordinator of the Assessment Unit of the College of Medicine. He is responsible for reviewing and approving summative assessment items before and after their implementation. In addition, he is a member of the secretary generals in the Progress Test Committee, which is responsible for planning and designing and implementing the progress testing at the levels of Saudi Arabian medical institutions on an annual basis, as well as a member of the curriculum steering and accreditation committees. His scholarly works center on student assessment, resilience and well-being, and curriculum development.

**M.wadi@qu.edu.sa**

**Mohammad H. Taha, MBBS, PG Dip, MSc (HPE), PhD** is Assistant Professor of Medical Education at the University of Sharjah's Medical Education Centre and College of Medicine, United Arab Emirates, with over 13 years of medical/health professions education and educational research experience. He is currently the director of the Medical Education Centre and the coordinator of the Master of Leadership in Health Professions Education at the University of Sharjah, as well as the chair of the College of Medicine's curriculum committee. Dr. Mohamed H. Hassan also is a member of several international organizations, such as the Association for Medical Education in Europe (AMEE) and The Network: Towards Unity for Health TUFH, and serves as a consultant for various undergraduate and postgraduate medical curricula in the Eastern Mediterranean Region (EMRO region). Dr. Mohammad H. Taha has authored numerous articles on curriculum development, social accountability, online learning, students' and residents' learning environment, and residency training.

# Chapter 1
# Basic Concepts

**Hosam Eldeen Elsadig Gasmalla**

**Abstract** In this chapter, basic concepts about the assessment are explained, starting with a brief historical overview. Then, types of assessment (formative and summative) and assessment methods (written and performance-based assessments) are outlined. Finally, the criteria that make an assessment good, including validity, reliability, cost, feasibility, educational impact, and acceptability are described in detail.

*By the end of this chapter, the reader is expected to be able to*

1. Define assessment, its types and methods.
2. Describe the criteria of good assessment, in terms of validity, reliability, equivalence, feasibility, educational effect, catalytic effect, and acceptability.
3. Comprehend "validity" as a unitary concept.

**Keywords** Assessment · Formative assessment · Summative assessment · Written assessment · Performance-based assessments · Validity evidence · Reliability · Educational impact · Educational measures

## Introduction

Assessment is the keystone in the universe of medical education. It requires using a systematic method for the collection of information to determine the candidate's performance/competency level [1]. George E. Miller stated that assessment drives learning [2]. Using this statement, we can extract that purposes and benefits from the assessment include encouraging students to learn, assessment is used for

H. E. E. Gasmalla (✉)
University of Warwick, Coventry, United Kingdom

Al Neelain University, Khartoum, Sudan
e-mail: hosam.mohammed@warwick.ac.uk


H. E. E. Gasmalla et al. (eds.), *Written Assessment in Medical Education*, https://doi.org/10.1007/978-3-031-11752-7_1

certification and judgment, it ensures attainment of the learning outcomes, and it is useful for program evaluation as it is crucial for monitoring the program.

The notion of assessment emerged more than 2000 years ago in China, during Hans's dynasty, and the purpose was to select people to serve in the government [3]. During the Islamic empire (medieval era), passing a test for competencies was mandatory to practice medicine, while admission into Jesuits priests' schools required competitive testing in the seventeenth century. In Europe, formal assessments were formulated in the eighteenth century in French and Viennese medical schools, and by the nineteenth century, the General Medical Council was established in the UK to oversee formal assessments in medical education. Assessment and medical education were then revolutionized in the USA in the early 1900s following the Flexner report [4].

The term "*Assessment*" refers to a process that involves testing, a systematic approach to collecting data about a measure, such as a competency [5]. While "*Evaluation*" is a broader concept that measures the value of educational programs or curricula. Unlike evaluation, assessment mainly focuses on a student or a group of students [6].

The term "*Assessment tool*" refers to the *type* of question that is usually used to assess students. Examples of some commonly used assessment tools include A-type MCQs (single correct answer) or R-Type MCQs (extended matching questions). The term "*items*" or "*test items*" refers to the units of the assessment tool in a particular test.

## Types of Assessments

Assessment types are evolved around two purposes: formative and summative, including other subtypes such as diagnostic and continuous assessments. The distinction between the types of assessment is easier to be based on the purpose. Summative assessment is judgmental in nature [7]. It is conducted for purposes of grading and certification, while formative assessment's purpose is to improve learning by providing feedback.

### *Formative Assessment*

Formative assessment has been considered as a distinct entity from summative assessment since the 1960s, and its notion has shifted from the context of program evaluation to be based mainly on the benefits of the learners, with the feedback being the central feature [8]. Formative assessment is conducted in-class [9], although some may consider adding an off-class, open-book format as a useful intervention as well [10]. However, this distinction between formative and summative assessment is not absolute. The purpose of summative assessment is "assessment of learning" mainly but with some "assessment for learning" in it, and the purpose of formative assessment is "assessment for learning" mainly but with some "assessment of learning" in it [7]. The system of assessment is based on a balance between both summative and formative assessments [11].

The benefits of formative assessment are underpinned by its features. In formative assessment, information about performance is collected and used meaningfully to enhance learning (especially deep learning) [12, 13]. It shifts the minds of students from focusing on just obtaining high grades on the final exam into engagement in learning and skills development [14]. Moreover, formative assessment promotes learning through constructive feedback [15]. Since the aim of feedback is to support learners to achieve the learning outcomes, it is a way to inform the learner about the gap between his/her current status and the desired learning outcomes, a comparison between the actual performance of the student and the desired standard [16]. Hence, formative assessment is considered criterion-referenced [17]. The importance of feedback is paramount, generally, better performance in formative assessments is associated with better performance in the final exam [10, 18], but even those students who have not got scores for success in formative assessment got benefit from feedback that helped them in their final examinations, and that was attributed to their active participation in formative assessment and making use of the feedback [13, 19, 20]. Furthermore, it is essential to follow-up to detect improvements in the learner's performance, which makes a formative assessment a process in which feedback is not the last element, but rather a part of a continuous cycle [21].

*Diagnostic assessment* is considered formative; it is conducted before the start of the course or training (before intervention) in order to obtain a need assessment. It is similar to the formative assessment; however, its timing implies its purpose: to adjust the educational process according to the needs of the learner.

## *Summative Assessment*

The purposes of summative assessments are the ranking of the learners, promotion, and certification. It provides feedback regarding the achievements of the learners and the accomplishment of the program objectives. Summative assessments take various forms, for example, final examinations, which are conducted at the end of a course, year, semester, and particular phase or level defined by the course outlines of the curriculum.

*Continuous or periodic assessments* are considered summative since the students' scores are collected and combined for the purpose of making a decision such as a pass/fail (scores are included in the final result) (Fig. 1.1).

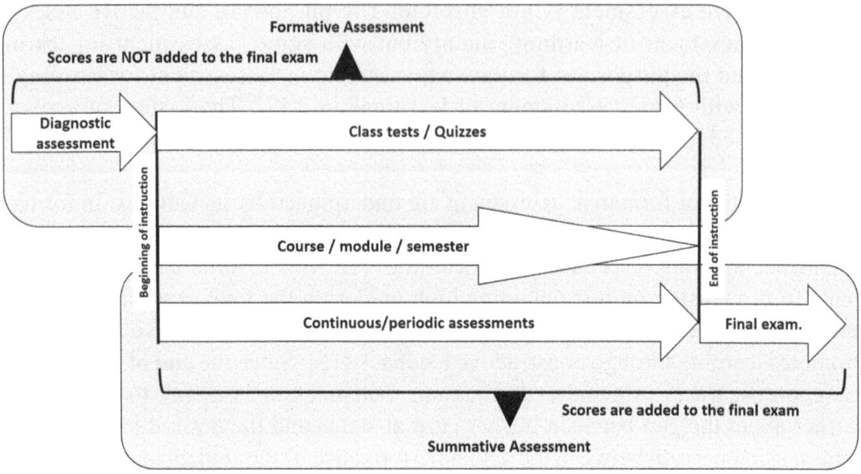


**Fig. 1.1** Types of assessment

## Assessments Methods

There are many ways to classify assessment methods based on the function of the assessment tools involved; Bloom's taxonomy demonstrates three domains of learning: cognitive, affective (attitude), and psychomotor (skills). Assessment methods can be classified according to the domain they assess, although the distinction is not necessarily sharp because some assessment tools in these methods can assess more than one domain.

### *Written Assessment*

This includes two formats of assessment tools. The first is the constructed response (CR) tool, in which the candidate writes down the answer. Assessment tools used in this method include essays and short-answer questions. The other format is the selected-response (SR), in which the candidate selects the correct answer from many other provided options, and assessment tools used in this method include the various forms of MCQs: the widely used A-type and R-type MCQs. The other forms of the selected-response are the true and false formats (C-type, K-type, and X-type). Written assessment can be introduced either in paper-and-pencil or computer-based formats (computer-based simulation).

## *Performance-Based Assessment*

Assessment tools used in this method can be classified into two groups, the first one is related to assessment in standardized or controlled conditions, it includes the well-known Objective Structured Clinical Examination (OSCE), as well as most of the simulations, such as standardized patients, model-driven simulation, and virtual reality [5]. (Note that computer-based simulation is used to assess knowledge and clinical reasoning, and since it does not assess performance and clinical skills, it is can be categorized as a tool for written assessment).

The other group of assessment tools is related to assessment in real situations known as a workplace-based assessment, including mini-clinical evaluation exercise (mini-CEX) and direct observation of procedural skills (DOPS) [22].

**Practical Application**

*Differences between "types of assessment," "assessment methods," "assessment tools," and "items"*

A formative assessment "type of assessment" can be developed to assess knowledge and skills using written and performance-based assessment "assessment methods," in which the utilized "assessment tools" in the written assessment part are A-type MCQs and modified essay questions, while the utilized assessment tools in the performance-based assessment part are OSCE.

A test consists of 50 "items" in which the "assessment tool" is A-type MCQs means simply the test consists of 50 questions in which the type of the questions is A-type MCQs.

**Take-Home Message**

*Types of assessment*

*Formative assessment*

Characteristics: conducted during the course/semester, in-class (mostly), feedback is a key feature. Scores are used for feedback and not collected for the final exam.

Purpose: to improve learning (especially deep learning).

*Summative assessment*

Characteristics: at the end of the course/semester (however, continuous assessment is considered summative in terms of including its marks/score in the final grades of the student). Scores are collected for the final exam.

Purpose: grading and certification.

*Assessment methods*

*Written assessment*

Constructed response (CR) (e.g., essays and short-answer questions)

Selected response (SR) (e.g., MCQs)

*Performance-based assessment*

Assessment in a standardized or controlled condition (Examples of assessment tools: OSCE, as standardized patient, model-driven simulation and virtual reality)

Assessment in real situations (Examples of assessment tools: mini-CEX and DOPS)

## The Quality of the Assessment

What makes an assessment good? There has been a consensus about the framework that makes an assessment good, including validity, reliability, equivalence, feasibility, educational effect, catalytic effect, and acceptability [4, 23].

However, in this book, we adopt the utility index introduced by Cees van der Vleuten, which includes validity, reliability, cost, feasibility, educational impact, and acceptability [24]. An understanding of the elements of this framework will help when planning or reviewing assessment programs to ensure that, wherever possible, all its components have been addressed adequately.

### *Validity*

The definition of validity has evolved over time. The current definition considers validity as a unitary concept; it is the degree to which evidence supports the appropriateness of the interpretations of test scores for the particular purpose of the test. The definition of validity has evolved from focusing on the validity of the test to the validity of its use for a particular purpose, and eventually, the validity of the interpretations drawn from test scores [25].

#### From "Types of Validity" to Sources of Validity Evidence

All "types" of validity, as well as reliability metrics, eventually share the same purpose of supporting the construct validity. Eventually, the idea of many "types" of validity was abandoned in favor of one unitary concept [26]. Therefore, the question of validity is as follows: are the interpretations and conclusions made by the teachers (about the competency level of the learners) accurate? Those conclusions (or inferences) need to be validated; this can be achieved by providing "validity evidence."

#### What Is a "Construct?

A "construct" is an intangible individual's characteristics; it cannot be detected directly. The behavior of the individual (exhibited as performance in a test) can be the only evidence of the existence of the construct. Thus, the construct can be inferred from the observation of the performance. As Cronbach stated, "*a construct is some postulated attribute of people, assumed to be reflected in test performance.*" Examples of constructs include clinical reasoning ability and communication ability, empathy, and professionalism.

**Practical Application**
*What is a "construct"?*

The ability to solve problems is an example of a construct. Validation includes posing test items (questions) to assess this ability. A common mistake is made during creating questions to assess problem-solving ability, by developing questions that focus only on the definition of the problem. Such questions require the ability to recall, which is a different construct than the one we intend to assess.

The specific behavior of the students is a "reflection" of a particular construct. This behavior can be manifested as a performance in the test. Thus, it is crucial to select the appropriate assessment tool, making sure that the questions represent a proper sample of the content [27]. Put in mind that each learning outcome is categorized according to the domains of Bloom's taxonomy: knowledge, attitude, and skills, thus, the assessment tool must be appropriate for the context of the domain.

## Sources of Validity Evidence

Sources of validity evidence can be obtained according to the following aspects: content, response process, internal structure, relationship to other variables, and consequences.

### Content

This aspect is concerned with the amount of evidence indicating that the test contents (including test items and instructions) represent the construct. An easy way to understand this is by asking three questions: what are the test items? (The answer in the blueprint), are those items of good quality? (The answer can be, as an example, in the forms for test revision), and who developed and revised the test items? (Their qualifications can be considered as the answer). Consequently, the evidence includes a blueprint (stating the cognitive domains assessed by each item), forms for test revision, and the qualifications of the test developers and revisors.

### Response Process

This aspect is about ensuring that the students respond to the test items according to the way those items were developed (i.e., the alignment between the responses and the construct). Evidence in this aspect answer queries such as: Did the student understand the questions properly? Did he/she know what to do to answer the question? And how to do it? Evidence in this aspect includes any documentation of the process of eliminating sources of error related to the administration of the test. It can be shown by providing and following a set of quality measures associated with test administration, such as instructions to the candidates, scoring process, and reporting of the scores. Security measures are also included.

### Internal Structure

This aspect is concerned with psychometric measures of test items, including aspects such as the reproducibility and generalizability of test scores. Evidence includes obtaining statistics such as item analysis (e.g., difficulty index, discrimination index, and distractors efficacy for MCQs). It also includes Cronbach's alpha (Kuder Richardson for dichotomous data) as an index of reliability.

### Relationship to Other Variables

State the correlations between this test and another one, the correlation is expected to be positive when both tests or assessment tools are investigating the same construct, and it is expected to be negative when they are examining different constructs.

### Consequences

This aspect considers the impact of the interpretation of test scores on the candidates and the educational process.

**Examples of Validity Evidence**

*Content*: Blueprint, test revision procedures and/or forms, and copy of the qualifications of the test developers and revisors.

*Response process*: Documentation of quality measures, such as instructions to the candidates, scoring process and reporting the scores, as well as security measures.

*Internal structure*: Statistics such as item analysis (e.g., difficulty index, discrimination index, and distractors efficacy for MCQs) as well as Cronbach's alpha or inter-rater reliability as an index of reliability.

*Relationship to other variables*: State the correlations between this test and another one or another variable.

*Consequences*: State the impact of the interpretation of test scores on the candidates and the educational process.

## What Affects Validity (Threats to Validity)?

To comprehend the concept of obtaining validity evidence, it is useful to examine the factors that negatively affect the validity (threats to validity), and overcoming those threats requires obtaining validity sources before, during, and after test development.

The test items must represent the construct; this requires developing enough test items to represent all the domains of the construct (i.e., ensuring proper sampling). Representative sampling is not confined to the number of items only, but it is extended to the domains, the test items must also represent the considered domains (cognitive, affective, and psychomotor) as well as the elements within each domain. If the cognitive/psychomotor domains ratio is 2:3, then this ratio would be the same in the test. This representative sampling can face some limitations. Limitation due to sampling is known as construct under-representation CU, or construct deficiency, and it includes developing few test items, which leads to under-representation of the construct, overrepresentation, and biased representation as manifested by mismatching between the test items and the construct, giving a clue to the students that specific topics are included (or excluded) in/from the exam, and focusing on certain domains (see Chap. 2: Assessment of Learning Outcome) while developing the test, whereas the test purpose requires the focus on all the domains in the specified area.

Another limitation (also known as construct-irrelevant variance CIV, construct contamination) includes disregarding the alignment between the learning outcome and the test items (e.g., using MCQs to assess psychomotor skills), introducing a test with item flaws or indiscriminating items and using an unjustified standard setting method. Overcoming this limitation is by avoiding item flaws, reviewing the test items before introducing them to the students, and selecting the proper method for standard setting.

**Practical Application**

*Overcoming threats to validity*

As a test developer, one must overcome the validity threats, the following steps can help:

1. Define the construct and its domains.
2. Develop test items ensuring proper sampling.
3. Select experts to revise the test items.
4. Review the test items.

From the mentioned steps, documentation is important, a blueprint can provide the best guidance for steps (1) and (2). In step (3), the qualifications of the experts must be stated/documented, while the process of revision in step (4) should also be documented (e.g., forms for test revision), all the mentioned documents are examples of validity evidence.

**Take-Home Message**

*Validity*

*What is it?*

Validity is a unitary concept; it is the degree to which evidence supports the appropriateness of the interpretations of test scores for the particular purpose of the test. Validation is an ongoing process of collecting evidence. In other words, it is the degree to which the interpretations of test scores are justifiable.

*Contemporary concepts versus old concepts*

*The shift from the validity of the test to the validity of the interpretations of test scores*

The definition of validity has evolved from focusing on the validity of the test to the validity of its use for a particular purpose, and eventually, the validity of the interpretations drawn from test scores.

*The shift from types of validity to sources of validity*

Evidence of validity can be obtained in relation to the following aspects: content, response process, internal structure, relationship to other variables, and consequences.

*Sources of validity evidence*

Sources of validity evidence can be obtained according to the following aspects: content, response process, internal structure, relationship to other variables, and consequences

## *Reliability*

It is the consistency of the results of the test (scores) in terms of the reproducibility of data. It also describes how precise the scores are in measuring performance and how much we can depend on the scores in drawing conclusions about students' competencies. Reliability is a property of the test scores and not the test itself [28]; for more understanding of the notion of reliability, let us think from a research point of view. The outcomes from any experimental study must be reproducible if the study is conducted again with similar conditions. Otherwise, the results cannot be considered reliable; using this concept, the assessment must yield the same results if introduced again to the same group of students.

### Why Obtaining Reliability Is Important?

Because it provides a source of evidence for validity. On the other hand, an unreliable test may result in the failure of a competent candidate, or the other way, the incompetent candidate may pass.

### What Affects Reliability?

Measurement errors can be related to candidate, assessment, or scoring process factors. Those factors are considered limitations to reliability.

To improve reliability, it is recommended to increase the number of items, in fact, this is an essential measure [28], other measures include avoiding item flaws and adopting objective approaches even when subjectivity is inevitable, and introducing a test in which all questions are too easy (or too difficult as well) can render the reliability low. However, high reliability can be obtained in some instances such as the bimodal distribution of the scores of the candidates; in this case, high reliability is not necessarily an accurate indication of the quality of the test.

### How to Measure Reliability?

There are many ways to measure reliability; in this chapter, we will focus on Cronbach's alpha, before that, it is useful to consider the following table (Table 1.1) for ways of measuring reliability.

**Practical Application**

*Cronbach's alpha*

*What is it?*

It is an index to measure reliability.

*When to use it?*

It is useful generally in selected-response tests (e.g., True/false and A-type MCQs)

*How to interpret it?*

It ranges from 0 to1. Below 0.5 is not acceptable.

Recommended range is as follows:

More than 0.90 for high stakes examinations.

0.80–0.89 for examinations at the end of the course/semester/year.

0.70–0.79 for formative assessments

*What affects it?*

The length of the test, a few test items drop the index.

**Table 1.1** Ways of measuring reliability

| The question needed to be answered | A suitable measure for reliability |
|---|---|
| Are all the items of the assessment tool measuring the same construct? | Split-half reliability<br>Kuder-Richardson<br>Cronbach's alpha |
| Does the assessment tool yield similar results when administered again? | Test-retest reliability |
| Do different versions of the same assessment tool yield similar results? | Alternate forms of reliability |
| How are raters agreed with each other?<br>(inter-rater reliability) | Percent agreement<br>Phi<br>Kappa<br>Kendall's tau<br>Intraclass correlation coefficient |
| What is the "error contribution" of each factor in the assessment process? | Generalizability coefficient |

**Take-Home Message**

*Reliability*

*What is it?*

It is the consistency of the results of the test (scores) in terms of the reproducibility of data; reliability is a property of the test scores and not the test itself. Reliability is one of the sources of validity, but it cannot stand alone as a sole source of validity.

*Examples of sources of reliability*

Internal consistency and inter-rater reliability.

*What is internal consistency and how to estimate it?*

If all test items are assessing the same construct, then there will be a consistency between them, and this is known as internal consistency. There are many ways to estimate the internal consistency, such as split-half correlation, and Kuder-Richardson and Cronbach's alpha indices.

## *Educational Impact, Acceptability, and Cost*

### Educational Impact

Assessment must have clarity of educational purpose and be designed to maximize learning in areas relevant to the curriculum. So, it should be designed according to the subject matter prioritization (see Chap. 2: Assessment of Learning Outcomes and Chap. 3: Blueprint in Assessment). The contents, formats, and programming of the assessment as well as the feedback of the results of the assessment are the four factors that underly the fact that assessment drives learning.

*Contents:* the contents of the assessment must represent the competency "or construct" that is needed to be assessed (e.g., for assessing problem-solving, it is useless to check recall in the test).

*Format:* the format of the test can affect learning; this includes the selection of the assessment tool.

*Programming of the assessment:* the timing and frequency of the assessments can shape the learning strategies of students; it also affects their level of preparation for each exam.

*Feedback of the results:* this can make the assessment a useful learning tool if provided to the students, it is also useful for the examiners and policymakers.

### Acceptability

The assessment must be acceptable for the teacher, student, and stakeholders. Faculty think about the impact of their experience on the judgment process on the candidates; they prefer direct contact with the student to assess them. Students are concerned about the fairness and clarity of the assessment tools and procedures. The public and stakeholders want to ensure that the assessment will yield the production of competent graduates.

### Cost

The better the assessment, the more it costs. Spending more on the assessment is beneficial for both teaching and learning; however, spending more can sometimes render the assessment impractical. Thus, it is a matter of balance.

**Criteria of Good Assessment and Validity Evidence**

Sources of validity evidence are content, response process, internal structure, relationship to other variables, and consequences.

The utility index (criteria of good assessment) includes validity, reliability, cost, feasibility, educational impact, and acceptability.

If we attempt to align both, it can be said that reliability is part of "validity evidence" under the *internal structure*. Cost, acceptability, and feasibility are part of "validity evidence" under the *response process*, while the educational impact is part of "validity evidence" under *consequences.*

So, it is all about validity after all.

## References

1. Schuwirth LW, van der Vleuten CP. General overview of the theories used in assessment: AMEE Guide No. 57. Med Teach. 2011;33(10):783-97.
2. Miller GE. The assessment of clinical skills/competence/performance. Academic medicine. 1990;65(9):S63-7.
3. Gipps C. Chapter 10: Socio-cultural aspects of assessment. Review of research in education. 1999;24(1):355-92.
4. Norcini J, Anderson B, Bollela V, Burch V, Costa MJ, Duvivier R, et al. Criteria for good assessment: consensus statement and recommendations from the Ottawa 2010 Conference. Med Teach. 2011;33(3):206-14.
5. Norcini JJ, McKinley DW. Assessment methods in medical education. Teaching and Teacher Education. 2007;23(3):239-50.
6. Gibbs T, Brigden D, Hellenberg D. Assessment and evaluation in medical education. South African Family Practice. 2006;48(1):5-7.
7. Bennett RE. Formative assessment: a critical review. Assessment in Education: Principles, Policy & Practice. 2011;18(1):5-25.
8. Ibrahim MS, Yusof MSB, Rahim AFA. Why Assessment Which Carries No grades and Marks is the Key for the Future of Education? Education in Medicine Journal. 2021;13(2):91-5.
9. Black P, Wiliam D. Developing the theory of formative assessment. Educational Assessment, Evaluation and Accountability (formerly: Journal of Personnel Evaluation in Education). 2009;21(1):5.
10. Krasne S, Wimmers PF, Relan A, Drake TA. Differential effects of two types of formative assessment in predicting performance of first-year medical students. Advances in Health Sciences Education. 2006;11(2):155-71.
11. Konopasek L, Norcini J, Krupat E. Focusing on the Formative: Building an Assessment System Aimed at Student Growth and Development. Acad Med. 2016;91(11):1492-7.
12. Al-Wassia R, Hamed O, Al-Wassia H, Alafari R, Jamjoom R. Cultural challenges to implementation of formative assessment in Saudi Arabia: an exploratory study. Med Teach. 2015;37 Suppl 1(sup1):S9-19.
13. Kibble JD, Johnson TR, Khalil MK, Nelson LD, Riggs GH, Borrero JL, et al. Insights gained from the analysis of performance and participation in online formative assessment. Teach Learn Med. 2011;23(2):125-9.
14. Dannefer EF. Beyond assessment of learning toward assessment for learning: educating tomorrow's physicians. Med Teach. 2013;35(7):560-3.
15. Rahman SA. Promoting learning outcomes in paediatrics through formative assessment. Med Teach. 2001;23(5):467-70.
16. van de Ridder JM, Stokking KM, McGaghie WC, ten Cate OT. What is feedback in clinical education? Med Educ. 2008;42(2):189-97.
17. Rushton A. Formative assessment: a key to deep learning? Med Teach. 2005;27(6):509-13.
18. McNulty JA, Espiritu BR, Hoyt AE, Ensminger DC, Chandrasekhar AJ. Associations between formative practice quizzes and summative examination outcomes in a medical anatomy course. Anat Sci Educ. 2015;8(1):37-44.
19. Carrillo-de-la-Pena MT, Bailles E, Caseras X, Martinez A, Ortet G, Perez J. Formative assessment and academic achievement in pre-graduate students of health sciences. Adv Health Sci Educ Theory Pract. 2009;14(1):61-7.
20. Velan GM, Jones P, McNeil HP, Kumar RK. Integrated online formative assessments in the biomedical sciences for medical students: benefits for learning. BMC Med Educ. 2008;8(1):52.
21. Dijksterhuis MG, Schuwirth LW, Braat DD, Teunissen PW, Scheele F. A qualitative study on trainees' and supervisors' perceptions of assessment for learning in postgraduate medical education. Medical teacher. 2013;35(8):e1396-e402.
22. Al-Wardy NM. Assessment methods in undergraduate medical education. Sultan Qaboos Univ Med J. 2010;10(2):203-9.

23. Norcini J, Anderson MB, Bollela V, Burch V, Costa MJ, Duvivier R, et al. 2018 Consensus framework for good assessment. Med Teach. 2018;40(11):1102-9.
24. Van Der Vleuten CPM. The assessment of professional competence: Developments, research and practical implications. Advances in Health Sciences Education. 1996;1(1):41-67.
25. Gasmalla HEE, Tahir ME. The validity argument: Addressing the misconceptions. Med Teach. 2021;43(12):1453-5.
26. Cook DA, Brydges R, Ginsburg S, Hatala R. A contemporary approach to validity arguments: a practical guide to Kane's framework. Med Educ. 2015;49(6):560-75.
27. Marilyn H. Oermann PDRNAF, Kathleen Gaberson PDRNCCNEA. Evaluation and Testing in Nursing Education, Sixth Edition: Springer Publishing Company; 2019.
28. Downing SM. Reliability: on the reproducibility of assessment data. Medical education. 2004;38(9):1006-12.

# Chapter 2
# Assessment of Learning Outcomes

**Alaa Abuelgasim Mohamed Ibrahim**

**Abstract** In health professional education, a learning outcome refers to a new skill, knowledge, or stimulus to improve the quality of patient care. This chapter explains what learning outcomes are and how to classify them. It also explains why it is crucial to think about learning outcomes when planning written assessments in medical education. In this chapter, different levels of the cognitive domains (Bloom's taxonomy), as well as the psychomotor and affective domains, will be discussed. Moreover, Miller's pyramid will be explained to help the reader think about how to plan for assessment more systematically.

*By the end of this chapter, the reader is expected to be able to*

1. Describe the concept of assessment of learning outcomes.
2. Describe Miller's pyramid and Bloom's taxonomy
3. Identify the suitable assessment tools for each cognitive domain.
4. Identify the most common types of written assessment.
5. Describe the differences between the most common types of written assessment.

**Keywords** Assessment · Bloom's taxonomy · Learning outcomes · Miller's pyramid · Validity

## Introduction

In health professional education, learning outcome *"refers to a new skill, knowledge or stimulus to improve the quality of patient care"* [1]. The curriculum includes a group of learning outcomes designed to achieve certain graduation competencies which are described as" *mastering of relevant knowledge and*

A. A. M. Ibrahim (✉)
College of Oral and Dental Medicine, Karary University, Khartoum, Sudan

Educational Development Center, Sudan Medical Spacialization Board, Khartoum, Sudan



H. E. E. Gasmalla et al. (eds.), *Written Assessment in Medical Education*,
https://doi.org/10.1007/978-3-031-11752-7_2

*acquisition of a range of relevant skills at a satisfactory level including interpersonal, clinical and technical components at a certain point of education,* i.e., *at graduation"* [2].

Historically, most educational institutes were using an input-based model for designing their curricula, which means throughout the curriculum they learn and then assess certain subjects to ensure the achievement of learning outcomes and thereby ensure occupational competencies. However, in the new era, curricula are designed based on a set of required competencies for mastering and safely practicing the desirable occupation. This design is called the outcome-based model. In this model, the occupational competencies guide the learning and assessment process through selecting the suitable learning outcomes for the achievement of the competencies. While the input-based model focuses on the process of teaching, the outcome-based model focuses on the outcome of learning and the impact of learning activities [3].

**Practical Application**

*Examples of competencies and learning outcomes*

*Competences*

Demonstrate application of history taking and clinical examination of the cardiovascular system.

*Learning outcomes*

Perform appropriately measurement of blood pressure using a sphygmomanometer.

## Outcome-Based Assessment

In the outcome-based assessment, the system of evaluation of professional accomplishments uses learning outcomes/objectives with certain criteria and standards as indicators based on the concept of outcomes-/competencies-based curriculum. This type of assessment is considered beneficial in many ways; first, by using the outcome-based assessment, we ensure the achievement of the desirable competence. Second, the assessment becomes more objective and structured for the learner and assessor by identifying what is expected from them at the end of the curriculum. Third outcome-based assessment is very useful in measuring the educational impact and predictive validity of assessment tools/items by predicting the actual performance of the learner in the real context. Finally, it justifies the criteria of assessment to learners and assessors. Outcomes-based assessment is considered a challenge because of lack of staff skill, required change of teaching and learning tools, time-consuming assessment, and the need for quality assurance systems [4].

**Take-Home Message**

*Outcomes-based assessment*

*Description*

- The system of evaluation of professional accomplishments uses learning outcomes/objectives with certain criteria and standards.
- Used mainly on outcomes-based curricula.

*Strengths*

- Ensuring the achievement of competencies and predicting future performance in practice.

*Limitations*

- Need training, quality assurance and time-consuming.

## Classifications of Intended Learning Outcomes

Many types of classifications and taxonomies are used in education to clarify domains and levels of learning outcomes. However, there are few types shown to be useful in the medical education field.

Benjamin Bloom with other educational psychologists divided learning outcomes into three domains of learning: cognitive (knowledge), affective (attitude), and psychomotor (skills) [5]. Bloom's taxonomy which was published in (1956) classified the cognitive domain to represent levels of reasoning of theoretical learning outcomes into six levels of reasoning from simplicity to complexity. In 1964, Krathwohl's taxonomy classified the affective domain to represent the levels of attitude and communications of learning outcomes into five levels of attitudes starting with a willingness and ending by adapting high professional values [6]. The third domain is the psychomotor, which was first classified by Simpson (1972) and represents the levels of skills and performances into seven levels from perception to creation [7]. Each domain and level have a preferable assessment tool according to the nature of learning outcomes thereby the written assessment tools (scope of the book) will cover only the levels of the cognitive domain.

**Practical Application**

Examples of intended learning outcomes ILOs for three major domains

*Cognitive domain*

Classify hypertension according to the best evidence-based medicine.

*Psychomotor domain*

Perform appropriate measurement of blood pressure using a sphygmomanometer.

*Affective domain*

Communicate appropriately with a patient before measuring his/her blood pressure.

## Levels of the Cognitive Domain (Bloom's Taxonomy)

As mentioned above, in 1956, Bloom divided the cognitive domain into six levels: knowledge, comprehension, application, analysis, synthesis, and evaluation which are rank-ordered from simple recall to complexity of judgment. Throughout 50 years, a lot of debate happened about the taxonomy ended with the recommendation of reversing the upper two levels and changing the way of thinking about the levels from outcome cognition to the process of cognition. In 2001, a group of cognitive psychologists revised Bloom's taxonomy and came out with a new six levels of processed cognition. *Remember:* which is the simplest form of cognition in which the learner is usually requested to recall or recognize the information. *Understand:* where the learner is requested to understand the meaning and consequences behind information or data, and the level is divided into seven cognitive processes (Table 2.1). *Apply* is a level when learners start to execute and implement their knowledge in real circumstances. *Analyze* is one of the high levels of cognition in which the learner is requested to make a deep analysis and interpretation of circumstances in the matter of critical reasoning, differentiating between elements, and organizing and deconstructing and quality of data. *Evaluate* is another level and the idea of cognition where the learner requested to make a judgment regarding theory or idea using critical appraising and evidence analysis. *Create* here the

**Table 2.1** Suitable examples of action verbs for use for each level of the cognitive domain [9]

| Cognitive level | Process of cognition | Action verbs |
|---|---|---|
| Remember | Recognizing<br>Recalling | Define, describe, identify, label, list, match, name, outline, reproduce, select, state, recall, record, recognize, repeat, draw on, recount |
| Understand | Interpreting<br>Exemplifying<br>Classifying<br>Summarizing<br>Inferring<br>Comparing<br>Explaining | Describe, estimate, explain, extend, generalize, summarize, clarify, express, review, discuss, locate, report, express, identify, illustrate, interpret, represent, differentiate |
| Apply | Executing<br>Implementing | Apply, change, compute, calculate, demonstrate, discover, manipulate, modify, operate, predict, prepare, produce, relate, show, solve, use, schedule, employ, intervene, practice, illustrate |
| Analyze | Differentiating<br>Organizing<br>Attributing | Analyze, diagram, classify, contrast, categorize differentiate, discriminate, distinguish, inspect, illustrate, infer, relate, select, survey, calculate, debate, compare, criticize |
| Evaluate | Checking<br>Critiquing | Appraise, argue, compare, conclude, contrast, criticize, discriminate, judge, evaluate, revise, select, justify, critique, recommend, relate, value, validate, summarize |
| Create | Generating<br>Planning<br>Producing | Compose, design, plan, assemble, prepare, construct, propose, formulate, set up, invent, develop, devise, summarize, produce |

**Table 2.2** Examples of learning outcomes of cardiac disease for different cognitive levels

| Cognitive level | Examples of learning outcomes |
|---|---|
| Remember | Define hypertension according to the best evidence-based medicine |
| Understand | Discuss the risk factors for different types of hypertension |
| Apply | Illustrate the common signs and symptoms of severe hypertension in emergency clinics |
| Analyze | Differentiate between clinical presentations of different cardiac diseases in the emergency clinic |
| Evaluate | Critically appraise the literature regarding different protocols of management of hypertension |
| Create | Design protocol for the management of hypertension in your local context using the best evidence-based practice |

**Table 2.3** Assessment tools for each cognitive level in Bloom's taxonomy

| Cognitive level | Suggested assessment tools |
|---|---|
| Remember | MCQs (A-Type) |
| Understand | MCQs (A-Type) |
| Apply | R-Type and A-Type MCQs |
| Analyze | R-Type and A-Type MCQs, constructed-response items |
| Evaluate | R-Type and A-Type MCQs, constructed-response items |
| Create | Constructed-response items |

learner is expected to construct, plan, and create new ideas and concepts that are processed from multiple sources and conditions to be represented in new circumstances [8] (Tables 2.1, 2.2, and 2.3).

## Psychomotor and Affective Domains (Tables 2.4 and 2.5)

**Take-Home Message**

*Bloom's taxonomy*

*Description*

Hierarchy of intended learning outcomes.

Cognitive, psychomotor, and affected represent the three major domains.

Each domain has different levels of reasoning.

*Strength*

Clarification of flow of information during the learning process and assessment.

Enhancement of student learning.

**Table 2.4** Practical examples related to the learning outcomes for each taxonomy: psychomotor domain

| Psychomotor domain | Action verbs for objectives | Example clinical learning outcomes |
|---|---|---|
| Perception: observation of behaviors involved in completing a task | Observe, attend to, ask, describe, participate, answer, detect, identify, differentiate, distinguish | Observe the correct technique for conducting a pelvic exam |
| Set: becoming mentally prepared to perform the task | The question, explore, consider outcomes, participate, tell, give examples, express confidence, begin, display, show, react, explain, move, state | Show the steps involved in conducting a rapid HIV test |
| Guided response: the early stage in learning a complex skill that includes imitation, performing a task with assistance, and trial and error; adequacy of performance is achieved by practicing | Complete, demonstrate, replicate, share, point out, break down, put together, copy, trace, follow, react, reproduce, imitate, respond | Demonstrate an IV insertion procedure safely and correctly on multiple patients under the supervision |
| Mechanism: the intermediate stage in learning a complex skill; learned responses have become habitual, and the movements can be performed with some confidence and proficiency (acting without assistance) | Arrange, choose, conduct, construct, design, integrate, organize, perform, modify, refine, vary, assemble, calibrate, construct, dismantle, display, fasten, fix, mend, grind, heat, manipulate, measure, organize, | Draw blood using universal precautions |
| Complex overt response: performing automatically with facility and habitually; fine-tuning and perfection of the skill or technique | Arrange, choose, conduct, construct, design, integrate, organize, perform, modify, refine, assemble, build, calibrate, construct, dismantle, display, fasten, fix, heat, manipulate, measure, mend, mix, organize, | Conducts a thorough physical examination |
| Adaptation: skills are well developed, and the individual can modify movement patterns to fit special requirements | Adapt, alter, change, rearrange, reorganize, revise, vary | Alter the patient treatment plan effectively based on the investigation results during the follow-up clinic |
| Origination: creating new movement patterns to fit a particular situation or specific problem. Learning outcomes emphasize creativity based upon highly developed skills | Arrange, build, combine, compose, construct, create, design, initiate, make, originate | Compose a comprehensive diabetic treatment plan based on the patient current condition |

**Table 2.5** Practical examples related to the learning outcomes for each taxonomy: affective domain

| Affective domain | Action verbs for objectives | Example clinical learning outcomes |
|---|---|---|
| Receiving (willing to listen): awareness, attention to new information | Ask, choose, describe, give, identify, locate, select, follow, reply, hold | Ask open-ended questions to elicit information during a patient counselling session |
| Responding (willing to participate): the active pursuit of an interest, willingness to respond, motivation | The answer, assist, discuss, greet, help, participate, present, read, report, select, tell, recite, label, perform | Present clients with risk reduction strategies appropriate to their needs |
| Valuing (willing to be involved): the worth or value a person attaches to a particular object, situation, or behavior; reflects the internalization of a set of values | Complete, demonstrate, differentiate, explain, follow, initiate, join, justify, propose, read, share | Demonstrate ability to provide a client with an HIV-positive test result in a compassionate and supportive manner |
| Organization (willing to be an advocate): the ability to prioritize and organize values | Adhere, alter, arrange, combine, compare, defend, explain, integrate, modify | Integrate professional standards of patient confidentiality into the personal life |
| Internalizing values (willing to change one's behavior): the ability to act consistently and predictably according to a value system or consistent philosophy | Act, display, influence, listen, modify, perform, propose, question, serve, solve, verify | Act objectively when solving problems |

## Miller's Pyramid

In 1990, another classification was published by George Miller, especially for competencies assessment [10]. The classification takes a hierarchical form base on the cognitive domain, while the top focus is performance and attitude in a four-level pyramid model. The base of the pyramid starts with the level of knowledge in the term "*Knows*" expressing the basic knowledge of information about competence, which includes the basic theoretical knowledge and understanding of the context of the learning outcomes to prepare the learner for the next level of the pyramid.

The second level of the pyramid expresses the application of knowledge in the term of *Knows-How*, in other words, how the competence can be obtained and in which circumstances. Here the learner becomes aware of the application of competence in a theoretical manner with a clear description of suitable clinical context and standard of application.

The third level expresses the demonstration of clinical skills competencies in the term of *Shows-How*. From here, clinical performance is the key competence, the learner watches, helps, and performs the desirable competence under supervision in a simulation or practical setting.

Finally, the fourth level expresses the performance of clinical competence in practice in terms of *Does*. Clinical context is the key to this level, the learner must select suitable circumstances to perform the desired competence in a clinical

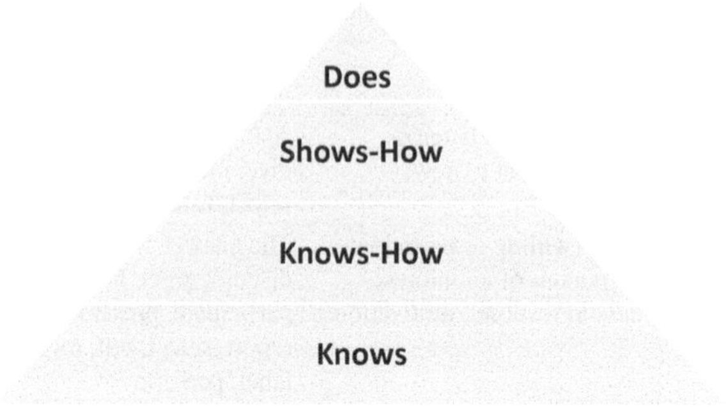


**Fig. 2.1** Miller's pyramid

**Table 2.6** Assessment tools for miller's levels of competencies

| Level | Type of assessment tools |
|---|---|
| Knows | MCQs |
| Knows-How | Essay-type questions/ extending matching questions/ case presentation |
| Shows-sow | Simulation/ OSCE |
| Does | Direct observation/ workplace-based assessment |

setting, including the patient's selection, clinical environment, and appropriate standard (Fig. 2.1).

Miller's pyramid is widely used in medical education, especially in the assessment of clinical competencies. As mentioned before, each level of the pyramid represents a different educational level thereby each level can be assessed with different assessment tools (see Table 2.6).

**Practical Application**

Examples of learning outcomes for each level in Miller's pyramid

*Knows*

List the types of instruments and materials needed for intravenous injection according to the best evidence of medical practice.

*Knows-How*

Describe the steps of intravenous injection according to the best evidence of medical practice.

*Shows-How*

Demonstrate intravenous injection in simulation according to the best evidence of medical practice.

*Does*

Perform intravenous injection in a clinical setting according to the best evidence of medical practice.

**Take-Home Message**

*Miller's pyramid*

*Description*

Hierarchy of competencies assessment
Four levels: (Knows, Knows-How, Shows-How, and Does)

*Strength*

Clarification of flow of information during clinical assessment
Easy to be used in health professional education

*Limitation*

Does not cover the high cognitive levels
Need modification to be used in clinical reasoning

## Types of Written Assessment

Questions of written assessment are classified under two main categories: constructed-response items (open-ended questions) and selected-response items (close-ended (multiple-choice) questions) [11].

### *Restricted-Response Items*

#### Commonly Used Multiple-Choice Questions

*Multiple-Choice Questions* such as *A-Type MCQs*: single best answer or single correct answer, the students choose one option (*key*) from 4 or 5 options, the rest of the options are usually referred to as (distractors). *R-Type MCQs*: or extended matching questions (EMQs): the students match given options with given scenarios, and the matching process is guided by a lead-in question.

*Assessed domain*: Any level of a cognitive domain below "Create."
*Strengths*: Grading is objective; these tools can introduce assessment of a huge amount of content, for a large number of students, in a relatively short time.
*Limitations*: Difficult to construct; students can answer by guessing and do not look authentic or strongly related to real situations.

#### Newer Formats of Multiple-Choice Questions

*Script-concordance* items are designed to assess the interpretation of clinical data in the context of indistinct or vaguely defined cases. In this type of question, a clinical scenario or situation is described, then a new finding is revealed, and the candidate has to assess the probability of a certain diagnosis or outcome in the light of this new finding.

*Key feature items* focus on critical decisions in particular clinical cases. It consists of three important components which are key feature details, key feature formats, and key feature problems. However, these items possess the characters of both the restricted-response items and constructed-response items.

## *Constructed-Response Items*

The basic value of open-ended questions is that the student is required to synthesize knowledge through retrieval and organization, while in close-ended questions, the student can find or recognize the answer from the provided multiple choices. examples for constructed response items; Modified essay questions and structured short-answer questions

*Assessed domain*: Mostly higher levels of cognitive domain and clinical reasoning.
*Strengths*: Students cannot answer by guessing, and higher cognitive functions can be assessed easily.
*Limitations*: Grading is subjective and time-consuming.

**Take-Home Message**
The content of the question is more important than its type and format in determining what the question tests.

## References


1. Wojtczak A. Glossary of medical education terms: part 4. Medical teacher. 2002;24(5):567-8.
2. Wojtczak A. Glossary of medical education terms: Part 1. Medical Teacher. 2009;24(2):216-9.
3. Harrison R, Mitchell L. Using outcomes-based methodology for the education, training and assessment of competence of healthcare professionals. Medical teacher. 2006;28(2):165-70.
4. Villaluz SS. Awareness on the advantages and disadvantages of outcomes based education among graduating Psychology students. Journal of Social Sciences (COES&RJ-JSS). 2017;6(2):224-34.
5. Forehand M. Bloom's taxonomy. Emerging perspectives on learning, teaching, and technology. 2010;41(4):47-56.
6. Krathwohl DR, Bloom BS, Masia BB. Taxonomy of educational objectives: the classification of educational goals; handbook.... 2. Affective domain: David McKay Company New York; 1964.
7. Hoque ME. Three domains of learning: Cognitive, affective and psychomotor. The Journal of EFL Education and Research. 2016;2(2):45-52.
8. Anderson LW, Bloom BS. A taxonomy for learning, teaching, and assessing: A revision of Bloom's taxonomy of educational objectives: Longman; 2001.
9. Chatterjee D, Corral J. How to write well-defined learning objectives. The journal of education in perioperative medicine: JEPM. 2017;19(4).
10. Miller GE. The assessment of clinical skills/competence/performance. Academic medicine. 1990;65(9):S63-7.
11. Epstein RM. Assessment in medical education. N Engl J Med. 2007;356(4):387-96.

# Chapter 3
# Blueprint in Assessment

**Alaa Abuelgasim Mohamed Ibrahim**
**and Hosam Eldeen Elsadig Gasmalla**

**Abstract** This chapter describes in simple steps how to systematically design and develop a blueprint for a test. It also provides several examples of different blueprints.

*By the end of this chapter, the reader is expected to*

1. Relate the importance of the blueprint to the validity argument.
2. Describe the component of the blueprint.
3. Create a blueprint for his/her assessment.

**Keywords** Blueprint · Validity evidence · Constructive alignment

## What Is Blueprint? Blueprint in the Context of Health Professional Education

In the context of health professional education, a blueprint, also known as a test plan or table of specifications, is a template that represents a systematically developed plan to ensure proper weightage and representativeness of contents and learning outcomes in the exam; enhance constructive alignment; and provide evidence of validity, considering validity as a unitary concept [1–3].

A. A. M. Ibrahim (✉)
College of Oral and Dental Medicine, Karary University, Khartoum, Sudan

Educational Development Center, Sudan Medical Spacialization Board, Khartoum, Sudan

H. E. E. Gasmalla
Al Neelain University, Khartoum, Sudan

University of Warwick, Coventry, United Kingdom



H. E. E. Gasmalla et al. (eds.), *Written Assessment in Medical Education*,
https://doi.org/10.1007/978-3-031-11752-7_3

## Theoretical Underpinning of Blueprint

Validity of the interpretations of test scores is backed by evidence. Blueprint stands as crucial evidence. It ensures the contents are represented properly (providing content-related source of evidence). It supports reliability through appropriate weightage of test items (providing internal structure-related source of evidence). The blueprint ensures conformity between learning outcomes, mode of delivery, and assessment methods and tools (constructive alignment). Thus, blueprinting is a cornerstone of developing assessments with high degree of validity of their interpreted scores [4, 5].

## Benefits of Blueprinting

**Systematic sampling** By including and weighing each topic/learning outcome in the course/ module and selecting the suitable assessment tool for each assessed learning outcome and domain, the blueprint links the assessment with the learning and teaching process and ensures constructive alignment.

**Providing validity evidence** As mentioned previously (Chap. 1), validity is an essential requirement in students' assessments. A blueprint is useful as a form of validity evidence [2]. Moreover, a blueprint guards against two threats to the validity [6]: construct under-representation (CU) (which occur when few items are used to cover the course material) and construct irrelevance variance (CIV) (which occurs when there are flawed item formats).

**Refining the curriculum** Another great role of blueprint is guiding the education process by selecting suitable educational experiences/ activities and reviewing the learning outcomes. Through the discussions regarding the agreed weight and importance of each topic/learning outcome, the development of the blueprint leads to a revision of the learning outcomes and helps the instructors refine and prioritize them.

**Quality assurance** Blueprinting is planning; it is a matter of quality. The blueprint document can be added to the required documents of the accreditation and quality assurance process. It serves as a clear map for assessors and provides a base for equitable and fair assessment and grading.

**Improving the perception of fairness** It was reported that publishing the blueprint to the students/learners enhanced their perception about the fairness of the evaluation process [4, 7].

**Developing a Q-Bank** Blueprint development helps in initiating and creating items for Q-Bank [5].

**Practical Application**

*When the blueprint should be designed?*

The blueprint should be developed after the curriculum has been designed and before starting the learning and assessment.

*Who should participate in designing the blueprint?*

The course/module creator includes content experts and health professional education experts.

## Designing the Blueprint

For designing an assessment blueprint, the following questions need to be considered:

**What is the purpose of the assessment?**
Formative or summative, the type of assessment influences decisions related to the sampling, depth, and types of questions in the exam, including the targeted domain.

**What is the weightage approach that you want to adopt?**
Approaches for estimating the weight of the contents include considering the importance of each topic/theme based on the estimation of the priority index [8], counting the number of contact hours of each topic, or weighing the numbers of specific learning outcomes. It is reported that there are no significant differences between those approaches [9].

**What type and level of learning outcomes do you want to assess?**
Define the domain of learning objective under assessment: cognitive, attitude, or psychomotor (according to Bloom's taxonomy). Identify the level of learning objective in each domain (e.g., for the cognitive domain: remembering, understanding, and applying). For the specifications of Bloom's taxonomy, please refer to Chap. 2.

**How do you want to assess it?**
Define the assessment tools that you want to use, usually, the assessment tool goes with the domain level of the learning outcome.

**How will you set the standards-setting for grades?**
Define the standard of grading either norm reference (according to peers' result) or criterion reference (according to preset criteria and quality). Stating this in the blueprint makes it a complete plan for the exam.

**Assessment's Blueprint**

**Department:** Physiology

**Course:** Cardiovascular system – **Code:** MED/123

**Assessment type:** Summative – end of course examination

**Total number of Questions:** 100

**Marking scheme**

**Total scores:** 100 assigned as follows:

| 50 A-type MCQs | 30 R-type MCQs | 20 Structured short answer questions |
|---|---|---|
| One mark for each | One mark for each | One mark for each |

**Pass mark:** 60

**Fig. 3.1** Suggested cover page of the blueprint

**Practical Application**

*Component of assessment blueprint*

For constructing a blueprint, many components need to be demonstrated:

1. Cover page (Fig. 3.1):

   The purpose of the assessment.
   Basic information: title of the course/level of candidates.
   Marking scheme: number of questions, marks of each question/group of questions, and total score

2. A table, worksheet, or spreadsheet describes the alignment between contents, learning outcomes, and selected type of questions (Table 3.6).
3. Plan for evaluation of the assessment.
4. Last page: stamps/signatures of the blueprint developers.

## Developing the Blueprint

In this chapter, we will describe the process of creating a blueprint based on the importance of each topic/theme according to the estimated priority index. There are six steps to develop a blueprint (Fig. 3.2) dispersed in two phases. The first four steps are included in phase one: topics' weights estimation. The fifth and sixth steps are included in phase two: selection of the appropriate assessment tool.

### *Phase One: Topics' Weight Estimation*

1. *Tabulate curricular content*

The first step in blueprinting is to define and tabulate the curricular content which is organized in a form of course themes, topics, or units. A blueprint template

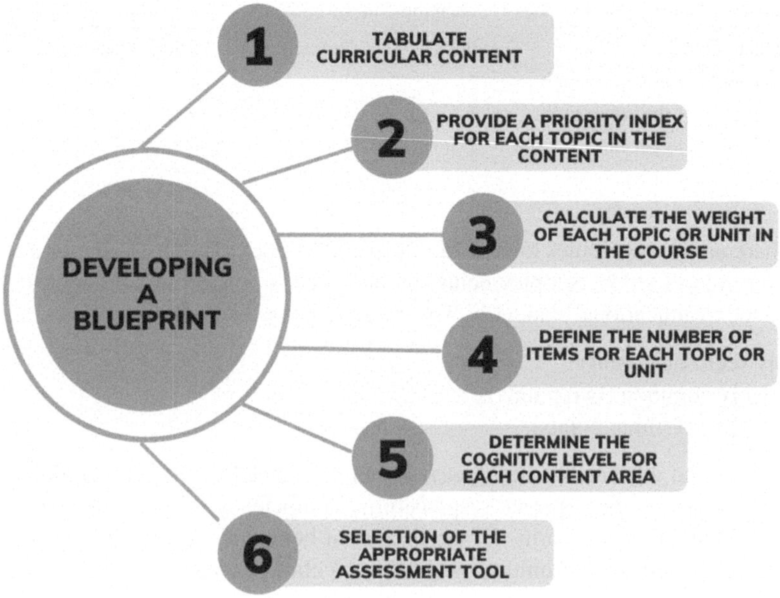


**Fig. 3.2** Six steps to develop a blueprint

**Table 3.1** Tabulating curricular content

| Anatomy of the musculoskeletal system I – Code: 122 / semester II | |
|---|---|
| Curriculum contents | |
| Blood supply of the upper limb | |
| Nerve supply of the upper limb | |
| Muscles of the upper limb | |
| Total | |

consists of a series of rows and columns (Table 3.1). At the head of each table, many elements need to be listed:

- Course title
- Student phase and level

2. *Provide a priority index for each topic in the content*

Assessment of the whole content of the curriculum is difficult. This highlights the need to set measures to ensure that every content area has an appropriate weight in the exam. This appropriateness should be measured by setting the priority index of each subject in the course.

**Table 3.2** Providing priority index for each topic in the content

| Presented topics | Impact | Frequency | Priority index (S × F) |
|---|---|---|---|
| Blood supply of the upper limb | 2 | 2 | 4 |
| Nerve supply of the upper limb | 3 | 3 | 9 |
| Muscles of the upper limb | 2 | 3 | 6 |
| Total | – | 19 | |

There are two attributes to measure the priority index. The first is the *frequency*. It is the rate of subjects/topics being applied/used in a specific field/context with reference to educational standards. The measure consists of a three points scale:

Rarely seen (one point)
Relatively common (two points)
Very common (three points)

The second attribute is the *impact*. It can be defined as the effect/influence of subjects/topics on the expected responsibility/competency of graduates with reference to educational standards. Or the burden of being "less competent, as a future doctor" on patients/communities' health for the clinical phase.

Low effect (one point)
Moderate effect (two points)
And high effect (three points)

Then multiply them together to calculate the priority index = frequency × impact. (Table 3.2)

**Practical Application**

*Priority index*

There are several ways to interpret "frequency" and "impact" according to the purpose of the assessment.

*Frequency:*

*One point:* rarely applied in phase two, or clinical practice, or rarely seen.

*Two points:* relatively commonly applied in phase two, or clinical practice, or seen.

*Three points:* very commonly applied in phase two, or clinical practice, or commonly seen.

*Impact:*

*One point:* less important for a medical student in phase 2, or a senior house office, or not life-threatening.

*Two points:* important for a medical student in phase 2, or a senior house office, or not instantly life-threatening.

*Three points:* very important for a medical student in phase 2, or a senior house office, or life-threatening emergency.

**Take-Home Message**

*Priority index*

*Description*

An index represents the appropriateness of the exam by ensuring its alignment and prioritization to the curriculum contents.

*Calculation*

The priority index = frequency of revisiting × impact of unknowing

*Criteria*

6–9 must know

3–4 should know

1–3 nice to know

*Toward objective judgment*

The selection of levels of frequency and impact is subjective. This can be improved by the involvement of two or more experts' opinions in the decision.

3. *Calculate the weight of each topic or unit in the course*

To determine the weight of the topic or unit concerning other curriculum content, first sum the priority index of the whole course contents then divide the item priority index by the sum of priority indices.

For example, the sum of priority indices for the anatomy of oral cavity course is 19. To identify the weight of the blood supply topic in the course we will divide the priority index of the blood supply to the sum of the priority indices of the course (4/19 = 0.21), which means that the weight of the blood supply topics in the content assessment tools should be 21% (Table 3.3).

4. *Define the number of items for each topic or unit*

The objective of the blueprint is to distribute the questions in the assessment tool according to their importance by applying the weight of every item or topic. Assume that the number of items is 10, then multiply it by the weight of a specific item in the curriculum. For example, the number of questions in (blood supply) topic = 0.21 × 10 = 2.1 questions (Table 3.4).

**Table 3.3** Calculating the weight of each topic or unit in the course

| Presented topics | Impact | Frequency | Priority index I × F | Weight: PI of item/ sum of PIs |
|---|---|---|---|---|
| Blood supply of the upper limb | 2 | 2 | 4 | 0.21 |
| Nerve supply of the upper limb | 3 | 3 | 9 | 0.47 |
| Muscles of the upper limb | 2 | 3 | 6 | 0.32 |
| Total | – | 19 | 1 | |

**Table 3.4** Defining the number of items for each topic or unit

| Presented topics | Impact | Frequency | Priority index I × F | Weight: PI item/ sum of PIs | The number of items: Item Wt. × total items No. |
|---|---|---|---|---|---|
| Blood supply of the upper limb | 2 | 2 | 4 | 0.21 | 2 |
| Nerve supply of the upper limb | 3 | 3 | 9 | 0.47 | 5 |
| Muscles of upper limb | 2 | 3 | 6 | 0.32 | 3 |
| Total | – | 19 | 1 | 10 | |

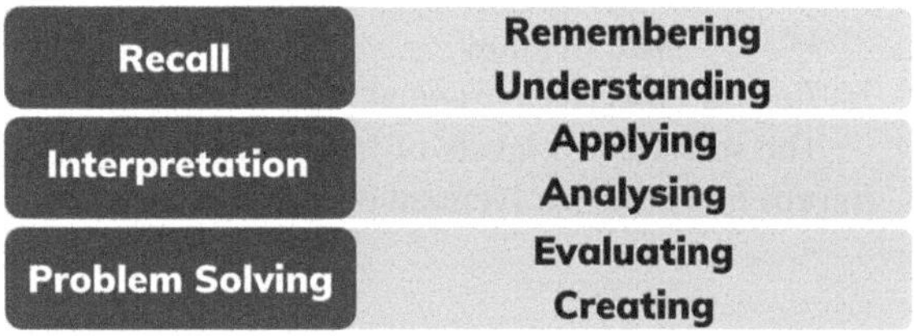


**Fig. 3.3** Grouping the six levels of the cognitive domain into three

Up to step 4, the number of assessment items for each course content is determined allying with their weights. The next step in the blueprint is to determine the type of assessment tools for each course content and according to their learning objectives.

## *Phase Two: Selection of the Appropriate Assessment Tool*

5. *Determine the cognitive level for each content area*

As mentioned in (Chap. 2), there are different levels in the cognitive domain. To practicality, the six levels of the cognitive domain are categorized into 3 categories (Fig. 3.3):

Each learning objective of the course should be categorized within those three categories of cognitive levels (Table 3.5).

6. *Selection of the appropriate assessment tool*

Each cognitive category has suitable assessment tools (see Chap. 2). In this step, the number of test items for each subject is distributed to a suitable cognitive category and thereby to their assessment tools.

The validity evidence for contents is now complete. Table 3.6, Figure 3.4 is the final step, and it is the suggested template to be included in the blueprint.

**Table 3.5** Determining the cognitive level for each content area

| Presented topics | Learning outcomes | Cognitive level |
|---|---|---|
| Blood supply of the upper limb | Describe the anatomical course of the arteries and veins that supply the arm, forearm, and hand | Recall |
| Nerve supply of the upper limb | Mention the roots, divisions, trunks, and branches of the brachial plexus | Recall |
| | Explain clinical picture associated with some nerves' injuries (e.g., a hanging, medially rotated arm, pronated forearm, and lost sensation down the lateral side of the arm in Erb-Duchenne palsy) | Problem-solving |
| Muscles of the upper limb | List the action of each muscle based on its origin, insertion, and course | Recall |
| | Describe the use of muscles of the upper limb in daily life (e.g., muscles used to open a cork or bottle of Pepsi, or in handshaking, or climbing) | Interpretation |
| | Explain clinical pictures associated with some muscles' malfunctions (e.g., weakness in the initial part of abduction and external rotation of the shoulder in rotator cuff tear, or abduction and external rotation of the arm in patients with anterior shoulder dislocation) | Problem-solving |

**Table 3.6** Selection of the appropriate assessment tool

| Presented topics | Impact | Frequency | Priority index I × F | Weight: PI item/sum of PIs | The number of items: Wt. × total items No. | Recall | Interpret | Problem-solving |
|---|---|---|---|---|---|---|---|---|
| | | | | | | A-Type MCQs, SAQs | R-Type MCQs SAQs | Problems |
| Blood supply of the upper limb | 2 | 2 | 4 | 0.21 | 2 | 2 | – | – |
| Nerve supply of the upper limb | 3 | 3 | 9 | 0.47 | 5 | 3 | – | 2 |
| Muscles of the upper limb | 2 | 3 | 6 | 0.32 | 3 | 1 | 1 | 1 |
| Total | – | – | 19 | 1 | 10 | 6 | 1 | 3 |

| Title/role | Name | Signature | Date |
|---|---|---|---|
| Developers | | | |
| | | | |
| | | | |
| Head of panel/committee of developers | | | |
| Head of the department/course coordinator | | | |
| Dean | | | |

**Fig. 3.4** Last page: stamps/signatures of the blueprint developers

## Examples for Blueprint Templates

### *Research Methodology Course (Table 3.7)*

**Table 3.7** Example for a blueprint for a research methodology course

| Research methodology Code: 326 / semester VI | | | | | | | | |
|---|---|---|---|---|---|---|---|---|
| | | | | | | Recall | Interpret | Problem-solving |
| Presented topics | Impact | Frequency | Priority index I × F | Weight: PI item/ sum of PIs | The number of items: Wt. × total items No. | A-type MCQs, SAQs | R-type MCQs SAQs | Problems /case studies |
| Research question | 3 | 3 | 9 | 0.1 | 10 | 6 | 3 | 1 |
| Literature review | 3 | 3 | 9 | 0.1 | 10 | 6 | 4 | |
| Research hypothesis | 1 | 2 | 2 | 0.023 | 2.3 = 3 | 2 | – | 1 |
| Research objectives | 3 | 3 | 9 | 0.1 | 10 | 5 | 4 | 1 |
| Study designs | 3 | 2 | 6 | 0.07 | 7 | – | 7 | – |
| Study population and area | 1 | 2 | 2 | 0.023 | 2.3 = 3 | 3 | – | – |
| Sample size | 2 | 1 | 2 | 0.023 | 2.3 = 3 | 2 | 1 | – |
| Sampling methods | 3 | 1 | 3 | 0.03 | 3 | 3 | – | – |
| Data collection methods | 3 | 3 | 9 | 0.1 | 10 | 5 | 4 | 1 |
| Designing of data collection tools | 3 | 1 | 3 | 0.03 | 3 | 2 | 1 | – |
| Ethics in research | 3 | 3 | 9 | 0.1 | 10 | 5 | 5 | – |
| Statistic in research | 3 | 2 | 6 | 0.07 | 7 | 5 | 1 | 1 |
| Proposal writing | 2 | 2 | 4 | 0.05 | 5 | 5 | – | – |
| Data collection and processing | 2 | 2 | 4 | 0.05 | 5 | 5 | – | – |
| Research report writing | 3 | 3 | 9 | 0.1 | 10 | 7 | 2 | 1 |

(continued)

**Table 3.7** (continued)

| Research methodology Code: 326 / semester VI | | | | | | | | |
|---|---|---|---|---|---|---|---|---|
| Presented topics | Impact | Frequency | Priority index I × F | Weight: PI item/ sum of PIs | The number of items: Wt. × total items No. | Recall<br>A-type MCQs, SAQs | Interpret<br>R-type MCQs SAQs | Problem-solving<br>Problems /case studies |
| Report printing and submission | 1 | 1 | 1 | 0.01 | 1 | 1 | – | – |
| Total | 39 | 34 | 87 | 1 | 100 | 62 | 32 | 6 |

## Conclusion

All assessments used in the course – formative and summative – should be prepared according to the blueprint. A well-constructed blueprint is a clear outline of the intended curriculum of a course. The details contained within a blueprint not only helps the course instructor to select appropriate content area but also helps teachers to plan the learning experiences so that the content delivered is compatible with both objectives and assessment. The blueprint should be provided for both teachers and learners to drive and monitor the educational experience, which ensures the concept of assessment drive learning.

## References


1. Messick S. Validity. In: Linn RL, editor. Educational measurement. 3rd ed. New York: Washington: Macmillan; 1989. p. 13 - 104.
2. Downing SM. Validity: on the meaningful interpretation of assessment data. Medical education. 2003;37(9):830-7.
3. Raymond MR, Grande JP. A practical guide to test blueprinting. Medical Teacher. 2019;8(41):854–61.
4. McLaughlin K, Coderre S, Woloschuk W, Mandin H. Does blueprint publication affect students' perception of validity of the evaluation process? Adv Health Sci Educ Theory Pract. 2005;10(1):15-22.
5. Coderre S, Woloschuk W, McLaughlin K. Twelve tips for blueprinting. Med Teach. 2009;31(4):322-4.
6. Downing SM, Haladyna TM. Validity threats: overcoming interference with proposed interpretations of assessment data. Med Educ. 2004;38(3):327-33.
7. Patil SY, Gosavi M, Bannur HB, Ratnakar A. Blueprinting in assessment: A tool to increase the validity of undergraduate written examinations in pathology. Int J Appl Basic Med Res. 2015;5(Suppl 1):S76-9.
8. Ismail MA-A, Mat Pa MN, Al-Muhammady Muhamad J, Yusoff MSB. Seven Steps to Construct an Assessment Blueprint: A Practical Guide. Education in Medicine Journal. 2020;12(1):71-80.
9. Salih KM, Al-faifi J, Abbas M, Alghamdi MA, Rezigalla AA. Methods of blueprint of a pediatric course in innovative curriculum. Onkologia i Radioterapia. 2021;15(8):1-4.

# Chapter 4
# Constructed Response Items

**Mohamed H. Taha**

**Abstract** Constructed response items (CRIs) are types of questions used to assess higher levels of the cognitive domain such as knowledge synthesis, evaluation, and creation. Many formats of CRIs are existing including long essay questions, short answer questions (SAQs), and the modified essay questions (MEQs). The aim of this chapter is to introduce you to CRIs' different formats, applications, their strengths and weakness, and how to construct them.

*By the end of this chapter, the reader is expected to be able to*

1. Discuss the different types of constructed response items' strengths and weaknesses.
2. Recognize how to create constructed response items.

**Keywords** Constructed response items · Open-ended questions · Essay questions

## Overview of Constructed Response Items and Rationale of Their Uses

Constructed response items/questions (CRIs) are part of written assessment methods that require the students to produce or construct the answer. Examples of constructed response items are the essay questions. CRIs have been used for a long period in health professional education due to several advantages including assessing the higher level of cognitive functioning, encouraging the students to think critically by forcing them to examine underlying facts, synthesize and propose new ideas, and justify their preferred option [1].

M. H. Taha (✉)
College of Medicine and Medical Education Centre, University of Sharjah, Sharjah, United Arab Emirates
e-mail: mtaha@sharjah.ac.ae



H. E. E. Gasmalla et al. (eds.), *Written Assessment in Medical Education*,
https://doi.org/10.1007/978-3-031-11752-7_4

Different formats of CRIs exist including long essay questions, modified essay questions (MEQs), and short answer questions (SAQs).

There is very little research on SAQs, particularly in medical education. However, research from secondary education suggests that CRIs such as SAQs can measure the same learning outcomes as MCQs if the stems are the same [2]. In the Netherlands, in medicine, SAQs have been effectively utilized as a trustworthy alternative to MCQ items in a progress test [3]. According to Palmer EJ et al. 2007, employing SAQ assessments can improve information retention over time compared to MCQ test [4].

On the other hand, CRIs have numerous shortcomings including relative lack of reliability and consistency in scoring. Furthermore, the scope of the question is not broad enough, as it tends to assess only a narrow amount of knowledge from the content and in this manner compromises the validity of interpretations. Testing for knowledge recall is a common misuse of CRIs, as it deprives them of their full power of assessing the higher-order thinking skills. This common misuse could take place by asking the students to list, mention, what......? [5]. Regarding the reliability and consistency of CRIs, it can be improved when using SAQs and MEQs.

Scoring of SAQs is one of the largest obstacles to the use of SAQs. They should be marked by experts in a reliable way and without inducing assessor effects (stringency vs. leniency) that confounds construct variance. However, there is much growth in intelligent computing making scoring of the items possible by computers, an idea first mooted in 1966 [6, 7].

## Types of Constructed Response Items

### *Long Essay Question*

Long essay questions have been used to assess complex learning situations that could not be measured by the other methods of assessment such as writing skills, the ability to present arguments succinctly. This format allows students greater flexibility in their response and reflects their unique approach, which can be evaluated in terms of interpretative skills [8, 9]. Several studies encourage the use of long essay questions due to the fact that writing necessitates a thorough comprehension of the subject matter as well as the application of cognitive abilities [10, 11]. Furthermore, it aids students in the development of higher-order thinking skills such as analysis, evaluation, and creation [4]. In contrast, some studies have concluded that the long essay questions are out of date because of low reliability and validity. However, it is still used in postgraduate medical education as written assignments [12]. Recently the long essay questions had been replaced by short answer questions and modified essay questions. Box (1) shows examples of long essay questions.

**Box (1) Practical Application**
*Examples of long essay questions*

1. Discuss the preventive measure of tetanus in different stages of life.
2. Professionalism is not only important as a characteristic of the doctor-patient relationship, but also with colleagues, the health care team, and hospital administration. Discuss this statement.

## *Modified Essay Question (MEQ)*

Modified essay questions are short clinical scenarios followed by a series of questions with a structured format for scoring. MEQs assess the student's factual memory, as well as cognitive skills such as information organization, clinical reasoning, and problem-solving.

MEQ is a unique form of essay question that comprises a case followed by a series of related questions. This leads to question interdependency, which means that if a student gets the first question wrong, he or she is likely to get the rest of the questions wrong as well [16]. Rather than assessing students' recollection of factual knowledge, a well-written MEQ evaluates their approach to solving a problem, their reasoning abilities, and their comprehension of concepts [17]. Recently MEQs are being phased out in favor of key feature questions due to psychometric issues with question interdependency [5, 18].

Key feature questions are short clinical cases or scenarios that are followed by questions that focus on the case's key aspects or important decisions [19]. Key feature questions have been promoted to test clinical reasoning and decision-making skills with demonstrated reliability when constructed according to certain guidelines [20]. Box (2) shows examples of long essay questions.

**Box (2) Practical Application**
*Examples of modified essay questions*

The patient is a 60-year-old Caucasian woman who presents to the emergency department with shortness of breath that started suddenly. Symptoms had started around 2 days prior and had progressively deteriorated, with no related, aggravating, or alleviating variables identified. She had comparable symptoms about a year ago that necessitated hospitalization. 20 Marks

1. What is your provisional diagnosis? (3 Marks)

   ……………………………………………………………………………………

   ……………………………………………………………………………………

   ……………………………………………………………………………………

2. Mention three of the first measures that should be performed by the treating ER physician (6 Marks)

.....................................................................................

.....................................................................................

.....................................................................................

3. List three important investigations that should be requested for this patient. (5 Marks)

.....................................................................................

.....................................................................................

.....................................................................................

4. Outline the first line of treatment for this patient in ER. (3 Marks)

.....................................................................................

.....................................................................................

.....................................................................................

5. What is the advice that should be given to this patient? (3 Marks)

.....................................................................................

.....................................................................................

.....................................................................................

## *Short Answer Question (SAQ)*

SAQs are CRI open-ended questions that ask students to develop an answer consisting of a few words up to sentences. The SAQ efficiently examined factual knowledge, which is vital for a doctor [13]. Only a small number of SAQs can be asked during an hour of testing time due to the time it takes to complete them. Before marking the question, it is critical that the questions are framed clearly and that an answer key is prepared [5]. The motivation for learning will be better when students are obliged to communicate their knowledge in the examination [13]. In CRIs generally, double marking is preferred if many examiners are available. However, each marker should correct the identical question for all candidates to save time. This produces more consistent results than if each marker corrects all of the questions for one group of applicants while another corrects all of the questions for another group [14]. The SAQs are considered more reliable than long essays but less reliable than MCQs because of the restricted sampling [15] Box (3) demonstrates example of SAQs and (Table 4.1) provides summary of different types, usages, design, advantages and limitations of SAQs and MEQs.

**Box (3) Practical Application**

*Examples of short answer questions*

Example [1]

World Health Organization guidelines for the diagnosis of diabetes recommend an oral glucose tolerance test if fasting plasma glucose concentration is in the range of 6.1–6.9 mmol/L. 10 Marks

https://www.who.int/data/gho/indicator-metadata-registry/imr-details/2380

1. What is the diagnostic term applied to patients with fasting plasma glucose concentration in this range? (2.5 Marks)

.......................................................................................

2. What are the consequences of this state for the risk of macrovascular disease and microvascular disease? (2.5 Marks)

.......................................................................................

3. What advice should be given regarding the management and follow-up of patients who fall in this category? (2.5 Marks)

.......................................................................................

## *Constructing SAQs and MEQs*

The construction of the SAQs and MEQs should follow a systematic approach as shown Box (4). This approach includes developing a blueprint and addressing the course learning outcomes. The learning outcomes are generally outlined based on Bloom's taxonomy including factual recall, comprehension, application, or analysis [21]. Higher levels such as creation or synthesis will probably require modified essay questions [22]. Then the item writer should state the item succinctly in plain, unambiguous language. A strong SAQs assesse factual knowledge as well as the ability to analyze and interpret a scenario clinically. It is good practice to give the student an indication of the length of answer required and to indicate how many marks are available for the question. Studies showed that positive perspectives (e.g., knowing the best method, describing good practice, or identifying the most relevant facts) have greater educational significance (e.g., in terms of the ability to measure objectives) than negative perspectives (e.g., knowing the worst method, unsatisfactory practice, or the least relevant issues) context [17, 18]. If you have to word an item negatively, it is advisable to use some form of emphasis for the negative words (e.g., "What is not an appropriate management option in this situation?"), using italics, bold type, or underlining to stress this for the test taker. It is worth mentioning that the item writer should try to avoid grammatical cues to the answer or providing answer spaces that are equal or proportional to the lengths of the required responses. Also, where a numerical answer has to be supplied, for example from a calculation based on clinical data, indicate both: a) the degree of precision expected (e.g., give

**Table 4.1** Summary of CRIs types, usage, design advantages, and limitations

| Type of essay question | Description | Usages | Construction | Advantages | Limitations |
|---|---|---|---|---|---|
| Short essay question—traditional | A single question, a short phrase, or a line or two of text is frequently all that is required to answer a short question. The answers are determined. | Specific facts or words about basic sciences or clinical processes can be recalled. The question provides context. | Construction is deceptively simple.<br>Can easily sample a large variety of knowledge domains. | Can be used in place of multiple-choice questions in situations where memory is deemed critical (e.g., decisions based on core knowledge and experience).<br>Automated scoring is becoming a reality. | There are numerous formats available, but little study on their application and psychometric features. This can result in cueing across things. |
| Modified essay question | Developed specifically for medical usage—primarily used in general practice. Case vignette with a strong framework, followed by questions on any aspect.<br>Concentrated on the management of a case or cases by candidates. Typically, the answer(s) are preset. | Concerns about clinical management. Some cue recognition and reasoning are required to make the connection between, for example, indications and symptoms and investigations and management. The question provides context. | Can readily transition from one stage of clinical management to another by addressing difficulties in slightly different circumstances, for example, patient management in one scenario and ethics in another. It is possible to do a more efficient sample of a broad area of knowledge. | Can be used instead of cueing. The question setter has influence over the context. Can necessitate a broad range of cognitive activities. | Careful design is required to avoid cueing. As a result, sampling knowledge across cases may be patchy. |

**Box (4) Checklist for review of constructed response questions Practical Application [24]**

1. Blueprinting: Does every question map to course learning outcomes?
2. Identify the specific learning objectives the item will cover.
3. Does every question target the higher level of Bloom's taxonomy of "apply" or above?
4. Does the model answer match the question?
5. Does the rubric match the model answer?
6. Does the rubric appropriately reward the application of knowledge over knowledge recall?
7. Does the item state what is required concisely in clear, unambiguous simple language?
8. Is the item aim clear? Does it state that one fact should have just one answer, and one aimed at alternatives (e.g., differential diagnoses) should have as many as are appropriate?
9. An indication of the length of the answer to indicate how many marks are available for the question is given to the student.
10. Is the item constructed for positive perspectives (e.g., knowing the best method, describing the good practice, or identifying the most relevant facts)?
11. Does the item avoid grammatical cues to the answer?
12. Does the item provide answer spaces that are equal or proportional to the lengths of the required responses?

your answer to one decimal place and answers within 5% of the correct value will be given credit) and b) that the appropriate units must be indicated [23–27].

## Using Rubric in CRI

The marking of open-ended questions is critical in order to maintain the validity and reliability of the test result; thus, adopting a rubric increases the rater's objectivity, and acceptable agreement among raters and reduces subjectivity. Due to the variety of open-ended questions included in this chapter, a separate rubric would be constructed for each modality: LEQs, SAQs, and MEQs. In the case of SAQs, a rubric may not be necessary if only one or two sentences are utilized and if the key answer to the particular sort of open-ended question with a model answer is provided. A rubric is strongly advised for lengthy essay questions, particularly those found in academic essays and postgraduate assignments. Table 4.2 illustrates an example of a rubric for an essay question.

## Key Feature Approach Questions

Another format of construct response items is the key feature items (KFIs). It consists of a short, clearly described case or problem and a limited number of questions asking essential decisions [28]. Such tests can consist of many different short cases, enabling broad sampling of the content and thus reliable test results per hour of testing time [28, 29]. Further description is provided in Chap. 5: Key Feature Items.

**Take-Home Message**
Every question format has its own set of benefits and drawbacks that must be carefully considered before selecting a question type. It is impossible to test all facets of a topic or competencies with only one sort of question format. As a result, using a range of different question formats is required to counteract the potential limitations associated with individual question formats, although constructed response items have their limitations, it has several advantages including assessing the higher-level cognitive functioning, encouraging the students to think critically by forcing them to examine the underlying facts, and synthesize and propose new ideas. It should be constructed according to the guidelines to improve its reliability and to present evidence of validity; faculty development is required to improve its qualities; designing marking criteria is critical; and marking should be done by two faculty members.

**Table 4.2** Example for a rubric used for students' admission in postgraduate entrance exams using long essay questions

| Areas | Unsatisfactory [1] | Marginal [3] | Satisfactory [6] | Good [8] | Excellent [10] |
|---|---|---|---|---|---|
| Relevance of contents | No relevant content | Few contents are relevant | Many contents are relevant, some irrelevant | Most contents are relevant | All contents presented are completely relevant |
| Structural relationship | No structural relationships are correct | Few structural relationships are correct | Many structural relationships are correct | Most structural relationships are correct | All structural relationships are accurately described |
| Writing | No organization or clarity, many serious grammatical errors | Little organization or clarity of writing, many grammatical errors | Moderate organization and clarity, some grammatical errors | Writing fairly well organized, good clarity, mostly grammatical | Writing well organized, clear, grammatical |

Assessor (1): ....................................Signature: ..........................................
Assessor (2): ....................................Signature: ..........................................

## References


1. Brown GA, Bull J, Pendlebury M. Assessing student learning in higher education. Routledge; 2013.
2. Edwards BD, Arthur Jr W. An examination of factors contributing to a reduction in subgroup differences on a constructed-response paper-and-pencil test of scholastic achievement. J. Appl. Psychol. American Psychological Association; 2007;92(3):794.
3. Rademakers J, Ten Cate TJ, Bär PR. Progress testing with short answer questions. Med. Teach. Taylor & Francis; 2005;27(7):578–82.
4. Palmer EJ, Devitt PG. Assessment of higher order cognitive skills in undergraduate education: modified essay or multiple choice questions? Research paper. BMC Med. Educ. BioMed Central; 2007;7(1):1–7.
5. Schuwirth LWT, Van Der Vleuten CPM. Different written assessment methods: what can be said about their strengths and weaknesses? Med. Educ. Wiley Online Library; 2004;38(9):974–9.
6. Swanwick T. Understanding medical education. Underst. Med. Educ. Evidence, Theory, Pract. Wiley Online Library; 2018;1–6.
7. Ramesh D, Sanampudi SK. An automated essay scoring systems: a systematic literature review. Artif. Intell. Rev. Springer; 2021;1–33.
8. Feletti GI. Reliability and validity studies on modified essay questions. J. Med. Educ. 1980;55(11):933–41.
9. Walubo A, Burch V, Parmar P, Raidoo D, Cassimjee M, Onia R, et al. A model for selecting assessment methods for evaluating medical students in African medical schools. Acad. Med. LWW; 2003;78(9):899–906.
10. Elander J, Harrington K, Norton L, Robinson H, Reddy P. Complex skills and academic writing: a review of evidence about the types of learning required to meet core assessment criteria. Assess. Eval. High. Educ. Taylor & Francis; 2006;31(1):71–90.
11. Kim S, Yang JW, Lim J, Lee S, Ihm J, Park J. The impact of writing on academic performance for medical students. BMC Med. Educ. BioMed Central; 2021;21(1):1–8.
12. Freestone N. Drafting and acting on feedback supports student learning when writing essay assignments. Adv. Physiol. Educ. American Physiological Society; 2009;33(2):98–102.
13. Puthiaparampil T, Rahman MM. Very short answer questions: a viable alternative to multiple choice questions. BMC Med. Educ. Springer; 2020;20(1):1–8.
14. Schuwirth LWT, van der Vleuten CPM. Written assessment. Bmj. British Medical Journal Publishing Group; 2003;326(7390):643–5.
15. Verma M, Chhatwal J, Singh T. Reliability of Essay Type Questions—effect of structuring. Assess. Educ. Princ. Policy Pract. Taylor & Francis; 1997;4(2):265–70.
16. Knox JDE. What is.... a Modified Essay Question? Med. Teach. Taylor & Francis; 1989;11(1):51–7.
17. Knox JDE. Use modified essay questions. Med. Teach. Taylor & Francis; 1980;2(1):20–4.
18. Al-Wardy NM. Assessment methods in undergraduate medical education. Sultan Qaboos Univ. Med. J. Sultan Qaboos University; 2010;10(2):203.
19. Bordage G. An alternative approach to PMPs. The" key Featur. concept. Further development in assessing clinical competence, Montreal Can-Heal ...; 1987;59–75.
20. Farmer EA, Page G. A practical guide to assessing clinical decision-making skills using the key features approach. Med. Educ. Wiley Online Library; 2005;39(12):1188–94.
21. Hamdy H. Blueprinting for the assessment of health care professionals. Clin. Teach. Wiley Online Library; 2006;3(3):175–9.
22. Hift RJ. Should essays and other "open-ended"-type questions retain a place in written summative assessment in clinical medicine? BMC Med. Educ. BioMed Central; 2014;14(1):1–18.
23. Sam AH, Field SM, Collares CF, van der Vleuten CPM, Wass VJ, Melville C, et al. Very-short-answer questions: reliability, discrimination and acceptability. Med. Educ. Wiley Online Library; 2018;52(4):447–55.

24. Hauer KE, Boscardin C, Brenner JM, van Schaik SM, Papp KK. Twelve tips for assessing medical knowledge with open-ended questions: Designing constructed response examinations in medical education. Med. Teach. Taylor & Francis; 2020;42(8):880–5.
25. Feletti GI, Smith EKM. Modified essay questions: are they worth the effort? Med. Educ. Wiley Online Library; 1986;20(2):126–32.
26. Downing SM. Assessment of knowledge with written test forms. Int. Handb. Res. Med. Educ. Springer; 2002. p. 647–72.
27. Patil S. Long essay questions and short answer questions. Mahi Publications, Ahmedabad; 2020.
28. Hrynchak P, Glover Takahashi S, Nayer M. Key-feature questions for assessment of clinical reasoning: a literature review. Med. Educ. Wiley Online Library; 2014;48(9):870–83.
29. Fischer MR, Kopp V, Holzer M, Ruderich F, Jünger J. A modified electronic key feature examination for undergraduate medical students: validation threats and opportunities. Med. Teach. Taylor & Francis; 2005;27(5):450–5.

## *Further Reading*

Downing, S. M. (2003). Validity: on the meaningful interpretation of assessment data. Medical education, 37(9), 830-837.

Downing, S. M. (2003). Item response theory: applications of modern test theory in medical education. Medical education, 37(8), 739-745.

Farmer EA, Page G. A practical guide to assessing clinical decision-making skills using the key features approach. Med Educ. 2005;39(12):1188–94.

Hift, R. J. (2014). Should essays and other "open-ended"-type questions retain a place in written summative assessment in clinical medicine?. BMC medical education, 14(1), 1-18.

Knox, J. D. (1989). What is.... a Modified Essay Question?. Medical teacher, 11(1), 51-57.

Knox, J. D. E. (1980). Use modified essay questions. Medical teacher, 2(1), 20-24.

# Chapter 5
# Key Feature Items

**Muhamad Saiful Bahri Yusoff**

**Abstract** The key feature (KF) items focus on the assessment of applied knowledge for clinical decisions and actions based on specific clinical cases. The key feature items are aimed at the critical aspects of a case in clinical practice or the actions most likely to cause errors that affect patient outcomes. This approach will best discriminate varying levels of competency from more competent to less competent examinees. KF items contain an adequate and representative sample of clinical problems and a scoring procedure that only rewards mastery of critical, challenging decisions or actions. The flexible response formats of examinations using KF items best fit the clinical task nature being assessed. This chapter describes the concept of KFs and the structure of KF questions (KFQs) and discusses evidence to support the validity of KFQs.

*By the end of this chapter, the reader is expected to be able to*

1. Define key feature items.
2. Describe the structure of key feature items.
3. Identify the psychometric properties of key feature items.

**Keywords** Key feature items · Clinical reasoning · Higher-order thinking · Clinical competency

## The Concept of Key Feature Items

Clinical reasoning is central to clinical competency [1, 2] and related to the thought process that occurs in clinical practice to guide decision-making and facilitate the assessment, diagnosis, and management of patients [3, 4]. Since clinical reasoning

M. S. B. Yusoff (✉)
Department of Medical Education, School of Medical Sciences, Universiti Sains Malaysia, Kelantan, Malaysia
e-mail: msaiful_bahri@usm.my



H. E. E. Gasmalla et al. (eds.), *Written Assessment in Medical Education*,
https://doi.org/10.1007/978-3-031-11752-7_5

is a fundamental component of clinical competence [1, 2], it needs to be assessed in health profession educational programs using valid and reliable tools [3, 4]. Examinations using key feature (KF) items are one such assessment method [1].

The KF-based examination was first introduced at a conference at the University of Cambridge in 1984 [5, 6] to replace patient management problems (PMPs) in the MCC's Qualification Examination based on the key elements in the resolution of any clinical scenario [4–8]. A key feature (KF) is defined as a significant step in the resolution of a clinical scenario that focuses on a tricky or critical aspect in the diagnosis and management of a problem, at which candidates are most likely to make errors [4–6]. In this way, it increases the validity and avoids sole reliance on multiple-choice questions for judging clinical competence such as clinical reasoning and decision-making [4–8]. The following are the three main characteristics of KF items [5–8]:

1. A critical or essential step(s) in the resolution of a clinical problem.
2. A step(s) in which examinees (in our case, graduating medical students) are most likely to make errors in the resolution of the clinical problem.
3. A difficult or challenging aspect(s) in the identification and management of the clinical problem in practice.

The development of a clinical scenario around KFs will facilitate a better discriminating measure of clinical competence such as clinical reasoning and decision-making [4–8]. The characteristics of KFs emphasize that not all steps in the resolution of a clinical problem are equally important and that testing time is better spent by concentrating on assessing the critical, essential, or challenging steps that define KFs [5–8]. It provides greater flexibility on issues of question format, multiple responses to questions, and scoring criteria. KF problems are designed to specifically assess clinical reasoning and decision-making skills rather than recall factual knowledge. While knowledge is a very important requisite for effective problem-solving, the challenge posed by KF problems is the application of knowledge to the resolution of a clinical problem—that is, the utilization of data to guide decisions to elicit clinical clues, to formulate diagnostic impressions, to order investigative or follow-up procedures, to accumulate data, to watch a course of action or evaluate the severity or probability of an outcome, or to pick a management course [4–8]. The nature of KFs will enable a better discriminating measure between competent and incompetent candidates.

Commonly, the label "KFQ" is used to describe a written test item that uses a context-rich clinical scenario that embeds KFs within the stem (a case description) and is followed by two to three questions [9, 10]. Typically, the case description is concise and includes relevant elements of the clinical scenario such as clinical signs and symptoms [11, 12]. The case description is usually presented in layman terms to minimize cueing with a limited number of questions per clinical scenario that focuses on KFs in the clinical scenario rather than recall of factual knowledge [11, 12]. These context-rich clinical scenarios require candidates to evaluate various information together to make clinical decisions or actions [10]. Interestingly, this KF format can even be incorporated into an objective structured clinical examination (OSCE) by developing an OSCE station around KFs of a clinical scenario [9]. Since its inception in 1992, four main benefits envisioned by the founders [5, 7]:

1. A broader sampling of clinical scenarios to increase reliability compared to PMPs.
2. More focused assessment of case-specific clinical decisions around KFs.
3. More flexible response formats to accommodate question types compared to PMPs.
4. Defensible pass-fail decisions.

The KF concept represents two important shifts from traditional positions in the assessment of clinical competence [5, 7]. First, it shifts the emphasis from the assessment methods to the assessment items [5, 7]. The first aspect to be addressed in developing a key feature problem is the selection of the clinical problem. This must be guided by and directly linked to the learning outcomes (competency). Once the learning outcome-linked problem has been selected, the next aspect is to tackle the critical, essential, or challenging aspects in the resolution of this clinical problem. The subsequent aspect is the method or methods that are best suited to measure the key features for this clinical problem. Thus, the assessment item is linked to the learning outcomes, and the methods are adapted to the item. Second, key features shift the emphasis from assessing all aspects of solving a clinical problem to assessing only the critical aspects relative to each clinical problem [5, 7]. This shift acknowledges that the key feature critical aspects in the resolution of a clinical problem are unique or specific to each clinical problem (known as "case specificity"). For some clinical problems, KFs may pertain to data gathering or interpretation while for others they might focus on selecting an appropriate therapeutic or follow-up plan.

## The Structure of Key Feature Items

KFs are usually unique to selected cases or presentations of a clinical problem, as they are going to vary relative to the clinical problem presentation and relative to other issues like the clinical setting, patient's age, and gender [5, 7]. Hence, it is uncommon to possess a "generic" set of KFs for a selected clinical problem. The KF problem format is attractive for assessing clinical reasoning and decision-making skills because they are relatively concise and concentrate only on a couple of KFs for resolving clinical problems. It is therefore allowing more clinical problems to be included on an examination within a fixed time (e.g., 30–40 KF cases compared to 10–12 PMPs during a half-day exam) [5, 7]. This wider sampling of clinical problems has direct implications to enhance the reliability of examination scores thus contributing to its validity. The KF format also allows a versatile approach to the question format, the option number to choose from, and instructions regarding the suitable responses to be selected. More specifically, the short-answer question format is available for situations where prompting/cueing from a list of options would compromise decision-making process measurement of candidates, or where listing options would provide too great support to weaker candidates, the individuals to whom the whole examination process is most frequently targeted [5, 7]. Eventually, the scoring keys are flexible for the number and configuration of correct responses to a question and may accommodate the complexity and configurations of conduct needed in the resolution of clinical problems [5].

KFQs consist of three important components which are key feature details, key feature formats, and key feature problems. Table 5.1 provides the key feature

**Table 5.1** Key feature details

| | | |
|---|---|---|
| Authors | XYZ | |
| Clinical problem | Age-related macular degeneration | |
| Learning outcome | Must be specified according to the assessment/ examination blueprint | |
| Patient age group | Paediatric (1-12 years) | |
| | Adolescence (12-18 years) | |
| | Young adult (19-40 years) | |
| | Middle age (40-60 years) | |
| | Elderly (>60 years) | X |
| Location | Ophthalmology clinic | |
| Clinical situation | Undifferentiated complaint | |
| | Single typical problem | X |
| | Multiple or multisystem problem | |
| | Visual threatening event | |
| | Preventive care and health promotion | |
| Comments | Critical knowledge<br>Optional coherence tomography (OCT)—Findings<br>Fundus fluorescein angiography (FFA)—Findings<br>Indocyanine green angiography (ICG)—Findings | |
| Patient's age | > 60 years old | |
| Patient's gender | Male | |
| Key features | Given an elderly male presented with progressive unilateral visual loss and macular edema with drusen, the candidate will | |
| | State the most likely diagnosis<br>Determine specific features of disease activity of the lesion based on appropriate investigations | |

[a]This case example was developed during the Malaysian Universities Conjoint Committee of Ophthalmologists (MUCCO) KFQ Development Workshop

**Table 5.2** Key feature format

| | |
|---|---|
| Case Scenario[a]:<br>A 75-year-old Malay male presents to outpatient clinic complaining of distortion and blurring of vision in the right eye for 6 months. He has no other complaints. He is hypertensive and smoker. He is not diabetic. On examination, visual acuity is 6/60 in the RE and 6/9 in the LE. Anterior segments were unremarkable. Fundoscopy showed submacular hemorrhage in the right eye with presence of drusens in both macula. Optical coherence tomography (OCT) revealed presence of subretinal fluid in the macula. | |
| Question 1 | What is the most likely diagnosis for this patient? |
| (Write-in format) | ______________________________<br>__________ |
| Key feature | State the most likely diagnosis |
| Scoring key<br>Score<br>1.0<br>0 | Criteria<br>Exudative/wet age-related macular degeneration (all components are required)<br>Other answer or more than 1 answer |
| Question 2 | What are the specific features based on appropriate investigations that determine the disease activity of the lesion? Select up to 3 |
| (Short-menu format) | CNV in B-scan ultrasonography<br>CNV in ICG<br>Leakage in FFA<br>Leakage in ICG<br>Polyps in ICG<br>Polyps in FFA<br>Subretinal fibrosis in OCT<br>Telangiectatic vessels in FFA<br>*OCT—optical coherence tomography; FFA—fundus fluorescein angiography; ICG—indocyanine green angiography; CNV—choroidal neovascularization |
| Key feature | Determine specific features of disease activity of the lesion based on appropriate investigations |
| Scoring key<br>Score<br>0.5<br>0.5<br>0 | Criteria<br>Leakage in FFA<br>Polyps in ICG<br>Other answers or more than 3 answers |

[a]This case example was developed during the Malaysian Universities Conjoint Committee of Ophthalmologist (MUCCO) KFQ Development Workshop

structure details to facilitate the development of a key feature question and it is strongly recommended to develop KF items based on the key feature details (Table 5.1). The common structure format of a KFQ is provided in Table 5.2, and the format for candidates to answer is provided in Table 5.3. There are two formats of key feature questions: write-in and short-menu. The write-in format requires

**Table 5.3** Key feature question for candidates to answer[a]

| | |
|---|---|
| A 75-year-old Malay male presents to outpatient clinic complaining of distortion and blurring of vision in the right eye for 6 months. He has no other complaints. He is hypertensive and smoker. He is not diabetic. On examination visual acuity is 6/60 in the RE and 6/9 in the LE. Anterior segments were unremarkable. Fundoscopy showed submacular hemorrhage in the right eye with presence of drusens in both macula. OCT revealed presence of subretinal fluid in the macula. | |
| Question 1 | What is the most likely diagnosis for this patient? |
| | ______________________________<br>__________ |
| Question 2 | What are the specific features based on appropriate investigations that determine disease activity of the lesion? Select up to 3 |
| | CNV in B-scan ultrasonography<br>CNV in ICG<br>Leakage in FFA<br>Leakage in ICG<br>Polyps in ICG<br>Polyps in FFA<br>Subretinal fibrosis in OCT<br>Telangiectatic vessels in FFA<br>*OCT—optical coherence tomography; FFA—fundus fluorescein angiography; ICG—indocyanine green angiography; CNV—choroidal neovascularization |
| (5 minutes) | |

[a]This case example was developed during the Malaysian Universities Conjoint Committee of Ophthalmologist (MUCCO) KFQ Development Workshop

candidates to provide answers, while the short-menu format allows candidates to select answers from the option list.

Based on several established guidelines [5, 7, 13] and the author's own experience with the training of KFQs development for clinical examinations, Table 5.4 provides 14 essential guidelines to facilitate the construction of good KFQs.

**Practical Application**
"The KFQ format provides educators with a flexible approach to testing clinical decision-making skills with demonstrated validity and reliability when constructed according to the guidelines provided." (Farmer & Page, 2005. Pg. 1188).

**Table 5.4** The 14 guidelines for constructing KFQs

| Areas | Guidelines |
|---|---|
| A. Key feature foundation | (1) In order to improve the validity of the test, the objective and domain of the assessment should be defined in as much detail as possible. |
| | (2) It is necessary to specify the context in which the items are to be used, which includes the population to which they are oriented and the circumstances in which they will be applied. |
| | (3) A key feature must fulfill at least one of the criteria:<br>A critical or essential step(s) in the resolution of a clinical problem.<br>A step(s) in which examinees are most likely to make errors in the resolution of the clinical problem.<br>A difficult or challenging aspect in the identification and management of the clinical problem in practice. |
| B. The expression of the domain and context in each assessment item | (4) The objective, domain, and context of interest should be the determining criteria in construction. Each item should cover a significant unit of this referent and form with the others test items. |
| | (5) Each item should clearly show the intended content. Both the syntax (i.e., arrangement of words) and the semantics (i.e., the meaning of words) should fit with those of the domain context of reference, without the addition of unnecessary difficulties |
| | (6) Once the items have been constructed, it must be made sure that they fit the domain and context of reference, especially as regard their distribution in the test. |
| C. The development of a key feature problem for each clinical problem by stated criteria | (7) Define the clinical problem situation for the case. |
| | (8) Define the key features of each problem. |
| | (9) Select a clinical case to represent the problem and write the case scenario. |
| | (10) Write examination questions for each case—in general one question for each key feature. |
| | (11) Select a suitable format for each question. |
| | (12) Develop a scoring key for each question. |
| | (13) Pilot test the problems to acquire test-item statistics to guide their refinement (optional). |
| | (14) Define the minimum pass indices of the problems using standard-setting procedures (optional). |

## Psychometric Properties of Key Feature Items

Psychometric properties of KFQs can be appraised based on the five main validity evidence categories which are content, response process, internal structure, relations to other variables, and consequences [6, 14–16]. The validity is central to enabling confidence in the use of any assessment tool, including KFQs. Most simply defined, validity is the extent to which the assessment measures what it is intended to measure, making the construct of clinical reasoning central to the notion of validity when considering examinations using KFQs [6]. The following are brief definitions of each validity evidence category [14, 15]:

(i) *Content*: Do assessment items completely represent the construct? The extent of a measure includes a specific set of items to reflect the content of the intended attribute to be measured.
(ii) *Response process*: Are assessment items completely understood by users? It is concerned with the relationship between the intended construct and the thought processes of users while developing/responding to the assessment items.
(iii) *Internal structure*: Do assessment items measure the proposed constructs? It is dealing with the degree of relationship between/among assessment items and constructs as proposed and commonly represented by reliability and factor structure.
(iv) *Relations to other variables*: Do assessment scores correlate with intended or unintended variables? It is concerned with the relationship of measurement scores with external variables measured by another instrument assessing similar concepts or a specific set of criteria. It can be represented in the form of convergent, discriminant, predictive, and concurrent validity.
(v) *Consequences*: Do assessment scores make a difference in reality? It is dealing with evidence regarding the significance of measurement scores of specific intended or unintended educational outcomes.

Table 5.5 provides a summary of the validity evidence sources to support the validity of examinations using KFQs [6, 17]. Each validity evidence category will be further elaborated and discussed in relation to examinations using KFQs.

## *Evidence Based on Content*

Do assessment items completely represent the construct? Evidence based on content (i.e., content validity) is the extent of a measure that includes a specific set of items to reflect the content of the intended attribute to be measured [14, 15]. The construct that the KF approach intends to measure is the challenging decisions that clinicians make when interpreting patient findings in a given clinical situation. It is not a measure of the clinician's reasoning per se, but the clinical decisions or actions are taken. The potential sources of evidence based on content [6, 16, 17] are presented in Table 5.6.

At least four studies reported that the examination blueprint was used as a primary means to assure content validity of examinations using KFQs [9, 18–20]. The following are several examples of KFQ examinations using the assessment blueprint to assure content validity:

(i) Content validity was assured in the RACGP certification examinations by blueprinting it to the International Classification of Primary Care Version 2 and a profile of presentation rates at general practices in Australia [18].

**Table 5.5** The potential sources of evidence to support the validity of KFQs

| Content[a] | Response process[a] | Internal structure[a] | Relation to other variables[a] | Consequences[a] |
|---|---|---|---|---|
| Examination blueprint<br>Representativeness of test blueprint to achievement domain<br>Test specification<br>Match of item content to test specification<br>Representativeness of items to domain<br>Logical/empirical relationship of the content tested to achievement domain<br>Quality of test questions<br>Item writer qualification<br>Sensitivity review | Student format familiarity<br>Quality control of electronic scanning/scoring<br>Key validation of preliminary scores<br>Accuracy in combining different format scores<br>Quality control/accuracy/ of final scores/marks/ grades<br>Subscore/subscale analyses<br>Accuracy of applying pass-fail decision rules to scores<br>Quality control of score reporting to students/faculty<br>Understandable/accurate description/ interpretation of scores for students | Item analysis data<br>1. Item difficulty/ discrimination<br>2. Item/test characteristics curves<br>3. Inter-item correlation<br>4. Item-total correlation<br>Score scale reliability<br>Standard errors of measurement (SEM)<br>1. Generalizability<br>2. Dimensionality<br>3. Item factor analysis<br>4. Differential item functioning (DIF)<br>5. Psychometric model | Correlation with other relevant variables<br>Convergent correlations—internal/ external (similar tests)<br>Divergent correlations—internal/external (dissimilar tests)<br>Test-criterion correlations<br>Generalizability of evidence | Impact of test scores/results on students/society<br>Consequences on learners/ future learning<br>Positive consequences outweigh unintended negative consequences<br>Reasonableness of method of establishing pass-fail (cut) score<br>Pass-fail consequences:<br>1. P/F decision reliability—classification accuracy<br>2. Conditional standard error of measurement at pass score (CSEM)<br>False-positive/negative<br>Instructional/learner consequences |

[a]These sources of evidence were adopted from Downing (2003)

**Table 5.6** Evidence based on content to support the validity of KFQs

| Content |
|---|
| Examination blueprint |
| Representativeness of test blueprint to achievement domain |
| Test specification |
| Match of item content to test specification |
| Representativeness of items to domain |
| Logical/empirical relationship of the content tested to achievement domain |
| Quality of test questions |
| Item writer qualification |
| Sensitivity review |

(ii) Content validity of the clinical decision-making component of the MCCQE1 was assured by examining practitioner opinions on the frequency of problems encountered in practice [19]. A focus on critical steps and a broad sampling of problems (36 cases for the MCCQE Part I) provide a foundation for the content validity of a key feature problem examination format.
(iii) Content validity of a modified electronic examination using KFQs with MCQs was assured by blueprinting the examination to the Swiss one-dimensional blueprint for internal medicine [9].

Educational research provides strong evidence for the content validity of KFQs [6]. That is, if such an examination is constructed from a carefully developed blueprint, it will consist of a representative and adequate sample of clinical problems from the domain of problems for which candidates are responsible. The questions within each problem will test only the important steps in its resolution. Flexibility in formats and scoring keys emphasizes the authenticity of this format and its ability to accommodate the realities and complexities of clinical medicine.

**Domain-test blueprint** The type of test blueprint used to select cases from the domain of interest will directly impact the specific KFs defined. For example, KFs will vary depending on patient age groups or patient contexts. Many types of examination blueprints have been selected on the following basis to define KFs [16]:

(i) Clinical disciplines (e.g., Pediatrics, Medicine, Surgery, Obstetrics-Gynecology, Psychiatry)
(ii) Clinical situations (e.g., undifferentiated complaint; single, typical, or atypical presentation; multi-system disorders; life-threatening event; preventive care; and health promotion)
(iii) Frequency or priority of problems in practice
(iv) Patient age groups from health services data
(v) Physician activities and dimensions of care

**Representativeness and adequacy of content tested to domain** For a test to have content validity, it must contain both an adequate and representative sample of cases from the domain of interest. Several studies have been conducted to verify the extent to which the content of KF-based tests represents the domain of interest [16]. Assessing candidates' decision-making skills for high stakes, patient safety, and quality-of-care cases is a domain of particular interest for credentialing agencies responsible for protecting the public.

**Quality of the test material** Test developers have made KF training and development guidelines available to item writers and staff to minimize construct under-representativeness and construct irrelevant variance [6, 16].

## *Evidence-Based Response Process*

Are assessment items completely understood by users? The response process is concerned with the relationship between the intended construct and the thought processes of users while developing/responding to the assessment items [14, 15]. The potential sources of evidence based response [6, 16, 17] are presented in Table 5.7.

Several studies reported positive evidence about the response process [4, 9, 18, 19] that was assured through various strategies as highlighted in Table 5.7. The following are a few examples of evidence about the response process to support the validity of examinations using KFQs:

(i) The Royal Australian College of General Practitioners (RACGP) certification examinations had shown positive response process evidence by candidates rating the examination to be at least adequate as a measure of clinical decision-making and 40% rated it as good or excellent [18].
(ii) When candidates taking the MCCQE1 were asked if the test questions were pitched at the correct level or were trivial or ambitious, 96% of respondents indicated that the questions were at the correct level [19].

**Table 5.7** Evidence based on response process to support the validity of KFQs

| Response process |
|---|
| Student format familiarity |
| Quality control of electronic scanning/scoring |
| Key validation of preliminary scores |
| Accuracy in combining different format scores |
| Quality control/accuracy/of final scores/marks/grades |
| Subscore/subscale analyses |
| Accuracy of applying pass-fail decision rules to scores |
| Quality control of score reporting to students/faculty |
| Understandable/accurate description/interpretation of scores for students |

(iii) One study that reported on the validation of modified electronic examination using KFQs administered with an examination using MCQs [9] indicated that candidates considered the KFQs to be authentic, problem-based, and interdisciplinary and that they represented a reasonable approach.

The response process of examinations using KFQs can be argued to be good when the examination is properly designed using a blueprint that captures the intended focus of the assessment. A variety of blueprints have been used, demonstrating the flexibility of the assessment format [4, 18, 19]. In a recent review of KFQs by Page & Bordage [16], the following are the 10 important pieces of evidence based on the response process:

(i) *Candidate familiarity with format*: To further minimize construct irrelevant variance in the scores, test administrators offer candidates opportunities to practice taking a KF-based test before actually sitting a live exam.

(ii) *Question and response formats*: A variety of question and response formats have been used with KF cases, from traditional multiple-choice questions (MCQs) and short-answer questions (SAQ), written constructed responses, to short and long menus, and oral questions. KF-based tests have also been administered as open- and closed-book tests. The KF approach is not a test or item format per se but an approach to assess challenging clinical decisions or actions likely to lead to errors in clinical practice. The choice of question and response formats for KF cases is determined largely by the type of decisions to be assessed and the circumstances in actual practice to achieve as authentic assessment of clinical decision-making as possible.

(iii) *Scoring rationale*: A unique attribute of the KF approach is that each KF may have one or more correct answers depending on the complexity of the challenge involved as is often the case in actual practice. This poses two scoring challenges:

1. Use of differential weighing of options within a KF, that is, giving different options different weights depending on the perceived relative clinical importance of each option.
2. Use of dichotomous or partial-credit scoring algorithms, that is, getting a score of 1 for having all the correct options for a given KF and 0 for missing one or more correct options versus getting partial credit for as many correct responses provided.

Negative marking is also not recommended, except when a negative action or decision is prescribed as part of a KF, such as ordering a potentially harmful and unnecessary investigation, or prescribing an inappropriate or contraindicated medication or procedure. Candidate errors can be categorized into three types: (1) failing to select any correct responses, (2) going over the maximum limit of responses, or (3) selecting a response that is inappropriate or harmful to the patient. They noted that by distinguishing among these types of errors, the accuracy of pass-fail decisions might be improved.

(iv) *Language used in clinical scenarios*: To maximize authenticity and construct relevant variance on a KF-based examination, one may consider the use of lay language instead of medical terminology in the clinical scenarios as would be the case in real life. Overall, the uniform use of lay terminology yielded the highest test score reliability, requiring 16 fewer cases and a third less testing time (29 cases) relative to the medical terminology condition (45 cases) to achieve a reliability of 0.80. The use of lay terms to describe clinical cases should continue to be encouraged.

(v) *Rater training and accuracy for write-in responses*: Calibrating raters' expectations are important to ensure the optimal level of inter-rater agreement. Furthermore, automated scoring has achieved superior inter-rater results, compared to previous human scoring and offers new time-saving and feedback resources to test developers. The inter-rater agreement through a standard scoring system can be improved by using global rating or checklist rating, In the case if there are extremes raters (i.e., low inter-rater agreement), it is recommended to simply average rater scores when there are multiple raters present.

(vi) *Quality control of final scores or grades*: In a spirit of full disclosure and transparency, testing agencies publish technical reports about the quality of their exams. For example, each year the MCC publishes a technical report that summarizes the fundamental psychometric characteristics, test development, and test administration activities of the KFQs and candidate performance on the examination, including validity evidence in support of score interpretation.

(vii) *Validation of test materials and preliminary scores*: Pilot testing, often with as few as 20 subjects, provides a means of verifying whether the test cases and questions are unambiguous and that the scoring keys focus exclusively on the KFs, and nothing else and thus can help minimize construct irrelevant variance. Both quantitative and qualitative information are collected from the test-takers regarding their time spent to complete the pilot test, level of difficulty of the items, acceptability, case and question formats, authenticity, feedback, technical issues, cognitive level tested, and clarity of instructions. Only when the test cases, questions, and scoring keys meet performance requirements, they are used as live items for scoring.

(viii) *Accuracy in combining scores from different formats*: The issue of combining scores from different formats occurs both within cases and across exam formats. As indicated in the previous section on question and response formats, combining scores from different formats does not impact generalizability. Results from a KF-based test can also be used on their own or combined with other formats or sections for an overall test score.

(ix) *Accuracy of pass-fail decision rule*: Various standard-setting methods have been used to set a pass-fail cut-off score such as the modified Angoff approach that includes candidate performance data to set a pass/fail cut score. In the Bookmark method, all the items in the test are ranked from least difficult to most difficult (using item response theory data) and each standard-setter then reads the items and indicates (bookmarks) at the point between the hardest question borderline test-takers (minimally competent) would be likely to answer correctly and the easiest question the borderline test-takers were likely to miss.

(x) *Quality of score reporting to candidates and institutions*: The accuracy of the results reported to candidates and institutions depends on careful test blueprinting and in large part on test score reliability and pass/fail decisions.

## *Evidence Based on Internal Structure*

Do assessment items measure the proposed constructs? The internal structure is dealing with the degree of relationship between/among assessment items and constructs as proposed and commonly represented by reliability and factor structure [14, 15]. The potential sources of evidence on internal structure [6, 16, 17] are presented in Table 5.8.

**Item analysis** Item analysis of individual KF scores can be used to flag items that are too easy or too difficult or nondiscriminating. The reason being either because of some deficiency or pitfalls in the case scenario, question formulation, scoring key, or because of actual performance levels among the candidates taking the test [16]. One study demonstrated that out of 10, eight KFQs demonstrated optimum discrimination index (0.31–0.63) and difficulty index (0.43–0.77) [21]. The best measure of case performance is the index of discrimination, that is, the ability of KFQ to best capture various levels of performance among the candidates taking the test. While there is no steadfast rule about an acceptable level of discrimination, Downing [22] recommends indices of at least +0.30 or higher. Negative

**Table 5.8** Evidence on internal structure to support the validity of KFQs

| Internal structure |
|---|
| Item analysis data |
| (i). Item difficulty/discrimination |
| (ii) Item/test characteristics curves |
| (iii) Inter-item correlation |
| (iv) Item-total correlation |
| Score scale reliability |
| Standard errors of measurement (SEM) |
| (i) Generalizability |
| (ii) Dimensionality |
| (iii) Item factor analysis |
| (iv) Differential item functioning (DIF) |
| (v) Psychometric model |

discrimination indices mostly indicate some misleading information in the KFQ. Analysis of item difficulty data can also disclose possible discrepancies between the perception of test-takers and their actual level of performance.

**Practical Applications**

(i) For a high-stakes examination, 25–40 clinical cases tested within 3–4 hours is optimal to achieve reliability of 0.75–0.90.
(ii) The recommended time for a KFQ is between 5 and 10 minutes.
(iii) Each KFQ is recommended to have 2–3 questions.(Hrynchak et al., 2014)

**Score scale reliability** Internal consistency (i.e. the consistency of scores achieved across the items included in the examination) was reported in six studies conducted in various settings to range from 0.49 to 0.95, with the majority at the upper end when 25–40 cases were used [6, 8, 9, 16, 18, 20, 23, 24]. Page & Bordage (1995) estimated the test length from test score reliability and found that 40 cases were needed to reach a 0.80 level of internal consistency, requiring 4.1 hours of testing time. In general, internal consistency of 0.70 to 0.95 (Cronbach alpha) has been reported as acceptable if sufficient cases are used (i.e., 25–40 cases) [6, 8, 9, 16, 18, 20, 23, 24]. The use of lay language over medicalese has been shown to improve reliability, and partial credit scoring systems produced higher reliability than dichotomous ones [4, 6]. However, these results should be interpreted with caution, as a low reliability can result from a low number of test items or from the effort to test heterogeneous constructs [12, 25]. The following are several factors that influence the reliability of KF scores:

(i) *Response format*. Page and Bordage, in a series of studies, developed a clinical reasoning assessment tool for the MCC. They also showed the reliability of an examination using KFQs to be influenced by test structure [4]. They demonstrated that short-menu and mixed-response (i.e., write-in and short-menu) formats have equal reliability, which tends to be higher than that of other formats. Single questions following a key feature stem had lower reliability estimates [4].
(ii) *Language*. Whether the examination was conducted in French or English did not appear to affect reliability [26]. In a study of how the use of lay versus medical language related to the accuracy of diagnosis on the KFQ component of the MCCQE1, lay language was found to result in the highest internal consistency and, as a result, required less testing time [27].
(iii) *Scoring systems*. Page and Bordage [4] also examined the effects of different scoring systems. They found that summed (the total of the question scores is the problem score) and partial credit (a score between 0 and 1 that reflects the degree to which all correct responses were made) scoring systems produced higher reliability than averaged (the average of the question scores is the problem score) and dichotomous (a score of 1 for providing a minimally acceptable

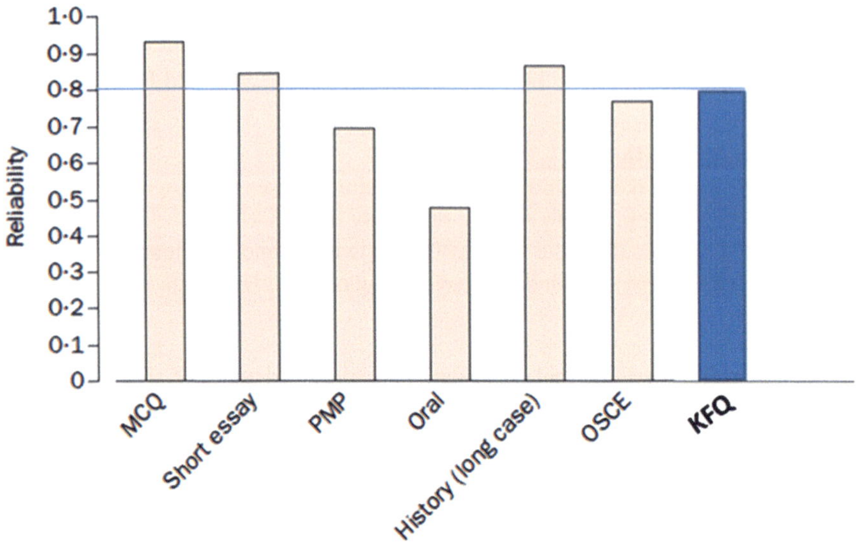


**Fig. 5.1** The reported reliability of different assessment methods when 4-hour examination time are used. (Adapted from Wass et al., 2001, pg. 946; MCQ multiple choice question, PMP patient management problem, OSCE objective structured clinical examination, KFQ key features question)

number of responses versus 0 for not providing the responses) systems. They also reported that the inter-rater reliability of write-in questions was 0.90 when physicians did the grading and 1.0 when computers were used [4, 6, 16].

(iv) *Test structure.* To determine more precisely which structural aspects of examinations using KFQs minimize the measurement error associated with this testing format, generalizability theory was used to parcel error variance into two parts: variance attributable to cases and variance attributable to differences between items within cases. As with all testing formats, case specificity is an issue that must be overcome: One study reported that 40 cases (which required 4.1 h of testing time) were required to produce reliability of 0.80 [4]. Another study revealed, however, that it is possible to optimize the reliability of examinations using KFQs by using two or three items per case rather than more or less [6, 28]. Figure 5.1 shows the reliability of KFQ in comparison to other assessment methods for a 4-hour examination [4, 29].

**Generalizability** Another approach to maximizing test score reliability is to conduct G and D generalizability studies to better understand the various sources of variance contributing to the scores and thus better design the exams [16]. The main source of score variance (30%) came from cases nested within these three factors related to disciplines, age groups, and clinical situations. Hence, it is important to construct KFQ examinations with large samples of cases (e.g., 40 cases), as each case makes a large independent contribution to score variance [4]. Out of these three factors, clinical situations appeared to be the more important factor to be emphasized.

The D-study from Norman et al. [28] showed that the optimal strategy in terms of enhancing reliability would be to use cases with 2–3 items per case. This finding has important practical implications for KF test developers, namely to prepare tests that contain a majority of multi-question (KFs) cases rather than single-question cases to maximize test score reliability; and limit the number of KFs tested to 2 or 3 per case because, beyond 3 KFs, no new information is contributing to the reliability of the scores and thus testing time is wasted.

**Item factor analysis** Factor analysis of the three main components of the MCCQE showed that the KF-based examination and the problem-solving portion of the OSCE occupied an intermediate position between knowledge (MCQs) and performance (OSCEs), which is in keeping with the accepted notion that clinical expertise involves both knowledge and other skills gained through experience. The results suggest that knowledge of broad disciplinary domains best accounts for performance on KF-based cases. In test development, particular effort should be placed on developing cases according to broad discipline and patient age domains. However, and by definition, KFs will vary depending on the clinical situation; for example, the challenging decisions related to managing chronic diseases are different depending on whether the situation is a life-threatening event in an emergency room versus an undifferentiated complaint during an office visit. Thus, blueprinting across clinical situations has its relevance.

**Differential item functioning (DIF)** DIF is a method used to determine whether test items behave differently for different groups of test-takers, such as candidates with different cultural or linguistic backgrounds. Early studies of possible French–English differences on the KF-based clinical decision-making portion showed that while there were 16% more words in French and the candidates took 8.47 min longer to complete the examination despite the high quality of translation.

## *Evidence Based on Relations to Other Variables*

Do assessment scores correlate with intended or unintended variables? Relation to other variables is concerned with the relationship of measurement scores with external variables measured by another instrument assessing similar concepts or a specific set of criteria [14, 15]. It can be represented in the form of convergent, discriminant, predictive, and concurrent validity. The potential sources of evidence based on relation to other variables [6, 16, 17] are presented in Table 5.9.

Examinations using KFQs intend to measure clinical reasoning and decision-making skills that utilize higher-order cognitive processes beyond simple factual recall. Evidence on relations to other variables is presented under three subheadings: convergent evidence (measuring similar constructs), divergent evidence (measuring dissimilar constructs), and test-criterion relationships [16].

**Table 5.9** Evidence based on relation to other variables to support the validity of KFQs

| |
|---|
| Relation to other variables |
| Correlation with other relevant variables |
| Convergent correlations—internal/external (similar tests) |
| Divergent correlations—internal/external (dissimilar tests) |
| Test-criterion correlations |
| Generalizability of evidence |

(i) *Convergent evidence*: Several studies using KFQs have shown that KFQ scores were highest for the group expected to have greater decision-making or problem-solving skills [16]. These results, and those from similar, provide convergent evidence that KFQs assess the construct of clinical decision-making.
(ii) *Divergent evidence*: Validity studies investigating correlations of KF-based tests with other measures show moderate correlations, typically in the 0.35 to 0.50 range [16]. These results raise the question of whether KF cases measure something different than other formats, especially in the sense of higher-order thinking beyond simple factual recall. More compelling than correlations are studies that use think-aloud strategies when comparing formats. This again supports the validity of KFQs as measures of higher-level cognitive processes. As measures of clinical decision-making, KFQs play a key role in helping to ensure that licensed and certified allied health practitioners have the skills they need to make important decisions on the job and improve their practice and quality of patient care.
(iii) *Test-criterion relationships*: How well do KFQ scores predict performance in practice? Tamblyn and collaborators conducted three studies that looked at the predictive relationship between MCCQ scores and complaints to medical regulatory authorities [30, 31]. They noted that KF-based clinical decision-making assessment was specifically designed to select problems and test aspects of the decision-making process where physicians were more likely to make errors that would affect patient outcomes and prompted them to suggest selecting cases and test questions for the problem-solving part of the OSCE-based clinical exam on the same basis as KF written problems. The KF-based clinical decision-making subscore was most strongly associated with the likelihood of receiving a complaint about communication or quality of care problems. Overall, the Tamblyn studies provide compelling evidence that KF-based test scores predict future practice.

Apart from that, four important findings highlighted by Hrynchak et al. [6] related to evidence based on relation to other variables. First, examinations using KFQs have been used effectively to measure the impact of educational interventions designed to improve clinical reasoning [1, 6, 16, 23, 24, 32, 33]. Second, experts have been found to do better than novices, and several authors have reported that examinations using KFQs can discriminate based on level of training [24, 34, 35]. Third, studies of divergent validity have shown that there is only moderate correlation between examinations using KFQs, MCQs, and clinical encounter cards [8, 9].

Fourth, a single think-aloud protocol study found that more complex descriptions of thinking patterns are used when solving KFQs relative to MCQs [36].

## *Evidence Based on Consequences of Testing*

Do assessment scores make a difference in reality? Consequences deal with evidence regarding the significance of measurement scores on specific intended or unintended educational outcomes [14, 15]. The potential sources of evidence on consequences [6, 16, 17] are presented in Table 5.10.

The scores, decisions, and intended, and unintended, outcomes of assessment can have a positive or negative impact on candidates, teachers, patients, and society [16]. Based on two recent reviews [6, 16], the following are the important highlights related to consequential validity evidence of KFQs:

(i) *Consequences on learners/future learning*: Fifth-year German medical students felt that, from an educational perspective, KFQs steered their learning toward clinical reasoning during their clerkships [16].
(ii) *Instructional/leaner consequences*: American medical students during their internal medicine clerkships preferred using the KFQ format for formative rather than summative purposes because they were reluctant to add an exam format specifically targeting decision-making ability that would count as part of the grade [16].
(iii) *Positive consequences outweigh unintended negative consequences*: One study examined physician performance as measured by incognito standardized patients (SPs) [35] and showed that examination results were not predictive of SP scores but did make it possible to differentiate between practitioners with more and less experience. The authors hypothesized that the SP scores were less valid because they focused on thoroughness more than on efficiency in data gathering. They concluded that the SP assessment technique had authenticity but not content validity and so was not a good measure of decision-making performance.

**Table 5.10** Evidence based on consequences to support the validity of KFQs

| Consequences |
|---|
| Impact of test scores/results on students/society |
| Consequences on learners/future learning |
| Positive consequences outweigh unintended negative consequences |
| Reasonableness of method of establishing pass-fail (cut) score |
| Pass-fail consequences: |
| (i) P/F decision reliability—classification accuracy |
| (ii) Conditional standard error of measurement at pass score (CSEM) |
| False-positive/negative |
| Instructional/learner consequences |

(iv) *Impact of test scores/results on students/society*: A study found that the clinical reasoning component of the MCCQE1 scores was highly correlated with physicians' future patients' adherence to anti-hypertension therapy [31]. The higher clinical decision-making scores were protective against nonadherence, showing that examinations using KFQs have predictive validity for future performance. The same researchers also looked at rates of complaint to the Colleges of Physicians and Surgeons of Ontario and Quebec and correlated the rate with the individual's previous results on the clinical reasoning component of the MCCQE1 [12, 25]. The complaint rate increased in a nonlinear way with decreasing score on the MCCQE1. This shows the predictive validity of the examination results in that they can predict future performance in the profession.

The paucity of consequential validity evidence of KFs [16] indicates further research should be done to provide more evidence to support it.

In addition to the five categories of validity evidence, Page & Bordage [16] highlighted additional two categories of evidence to support the validity of KFQs which are evidence on cost-feasibility and acceptability.

(i) *Evidence on cost and feasibility*: The development and maintenance of KF examinations are costly in time and resources because the KF-based test preparation is very labor-intensive. It takes a lot of time to produce a good case, and the key decisions are often difficult to define. It was estimated that it takes about 2 to 3 hours to develop and review a KF case by experienced item writers. However, as the case writers gain experience, the production time decreases to some extent. Similarly, administering a high-stakes KF-based examination via the internet found that the web-based format allowed us to administer the test to multiple sites easily and automated the marking of the examination. At present, short case-based assessment is being used with more success like KF cases. Although the KF-based examination is work-intensive, its widespread use to assess clinical decision-making skills provides evidence of its feasibility. The use of automated scoring of KF write-in questions is the way to improve consistency of scoring (i.e., efficiency) while reducing cost (i.e., time required for scoring and reporting).

(ii) *Evidence based on acceptability*: Acceptability refers to stakeholders finding the assessment process and results to be credible. Candidates taking a KF-based test from various countries (Australia, Canada, Germany, and the United States) concur that KF-based tests are credible, including the process and format, the authenticity and relevance of the cases, and the decision-making competencies tested.

## Conclusion

The key feature approach to assessment was proposed as a more efficient and effective means of assessing clinical decision-making skills. KFQs provide a greater flexibility to medical teachers to construct an effective assessment item to assess the clinical reasoning and decision-making skills of candidates. KFQs show many evidence to support its validity for assessing the clinical reasoning and decision-making skills. Hence, KFQ is the recommended assessment method for the assessment of the clinical reasoning and decision-making skills because it is valid, reliable, feasible, and cost-effective. While one set of articles reported meeting the validity standards, another set examined KF test development choices and score interpretation. The accumulated validity evidence for the KF approach since its inception supports the decision-making construct measured and its use to assess clinical decision-making skills at all levels of training and practice and with various types of exam formats. There are some areas with limited evidence, such as relations of KF scores to other variables, consequences of testing and its use for formative or programmatic assessment. These gaps push the KF approach forward and call for new research and validation studies.

## References

1. Daniel M, Rencic J, Durning SJ, Holmboe E, Santen SA, Lang V, et al. Clinical Reasoning Assessment Methods: A Scoping Review and Practical Guidance [Internet]. Vol. 94, Academic Medicine. Lippincott Williams and Wilkins; 2019 [cited 2021 Nov 27]. p. 902–12. Available from: https://journals.lww.com/academicmedicine/Fulltext/2019/06000/Clinical_Reasoning_Assessment_Methods__A_Scoping.52.aspx
2. Cumming A, Ross M. The Tuning Project for medicine - Learning outcomes for undergraduate medical education in Europe. Med Teach [Internet]. 2007 Sep [cited 2021 Nov 27];29(7):636–41. Available from: https://www.tandfonline.com/doi/abs/10.1080/01421590701721721
3. Lee CY, Jenq CC, Chandratilake M, Chen J, Chen MM, Nishigori H, et al. A scoping review of clinical reasoning research with Asian healthcare professionals. Adv Heal Sci Educ. 2021;26(2021):1555–79.
4. Page G, Bordage G. The medical council of Canada's key features project: A more valid written examination of clinical decision-making skills. Acad Med [Internet]. 1995 [cited 2021 Nov 24];70(2):104–10. Available from: https://europepmc.org/article/med/7865034
5. Medical Council of Canada. Guidelines for the Development of Key Feature Problems & Test Cases [Internet]. Vol. 2012. 2012 [cited 2021 Nov 24]. Available from: https://scholar.google.com/scholar?hl=en&as_sdt=0%2C5&q=Guidelines+For+The+Development+Of+Key+Feature+Problems+%26+Test+Cases&btnG=
6. Hrynchak P, Glover Takahashi S, Nayer M. Key-feature questions for assessment of clinical reasoning: A literature review. Med Educ. 2014;48(9):870–83.
7. Page G, Bordage G, Allen T. Developing key-feature problems and examinations to assess clinical decision-making skills. Acad Med [Internet]. 1995 [cited 2021 Nov 24];70(3):194–201. Available from: https://www.academia.edu/download/42782335/Developing_Key-Feature_Problems_and_Exam20160217-29772-12wzshl.pdf

8. Hatala R, Norman GR. Adapting the Key Features Examination for a clinical clerkship. Med Educ. 2002;36(2):160–5.
9. Fischer MR, Kopp V, Holzer M, Ruderich F, Jünger J. A modified electronic key feature examination for undergraduate medical students: Validation threats and opportunities. Med Teach [Internet]. 2005 Aug [cited 2021 Nov 24];27(5):450–5. Available from: https://www.tandfonline.com/doi/abs/10.1080/01421590500078471?casa_token=4jrVOtFGMS4AAAAA:lB2LHXGzO6HuYa1zIP_HifwiZ-28lcsUn9KqUAaS8_nXEhe-5QX05bJ_SHsh4KKV6U-Ug9x_FrHlug
10. Schuwirth LWT, Van Der Vleuten CPM. Different written assessment methods: What can be said about their strengths and weakness? Med Educ. 2004 Sep;38(9):974–9.
11. Haynes AB, Weiser TG, Berry WR, Lipsitz SR, Breizat A-HS, Dellinger EP, et al. A Surgical Safety Checklist to Reduce Morbidity and Mortality in a Global Population. N Engl J Med. 2009 Jan 29;360(5):491–9.
12. Tavakol M, Dennick R. Making sense of Cronbach's alpha [Internet]. Vol. 2, International Journal of Medical Education. IJME; 2011 [cited 2021 Nov 24]. p. 53–5. Available from: /pmc/articles/PMC4205511/
13. Farmer EA, Page G. A practical guide to assessing clinical decision-making skills using the key features approach. Med Educ. 2005 Dec;39(12):1188–94.
14. Cook DA, Beckman TJ. Current concepts in validity and reliability for psychometric instruments: theory and application. Am J Med. 2006;119(2):166.e7-16.
15. Yusoff MSB. A systematic review on validity evidence of medical student stressor questionnaire. Educ Med J. 2017;9(1):1–16.
16. Bordage G, Page G. The key-features approach to assess clinical decisions: validity evidence to date [Internet]. Vol. 23, Advances in Health Sciences Education. Springer Netherlands; 2018 [cited 2021 Nov 26]. p. 1005–36. Available from: https://link.springer.com/article/10.1007/s10459-018-9830-5
17. Downing SM. Validity: On the meaningful interpretation of assessment data. Vol. 37, Medical Education. 2003. p. 830–7.
18. Farmer E, Hinchy J. Assessing general practice clinical decision-making skills: the key feature approach. Aust Fam Physician. 2005;34(12):1059–61.
19. Bordage G, Brailovsky C, Carretier H, Page G. Content validation of key features on a national examination of clinical decision-Making skills. Acad Med [Internet]. 1995 [cited 2021 Nov 24];70(4):276–81. Available from: https://psycnet.apa.org/record/1995-42524-001
20. Trudel J, Bordage G, Sowing S. Reliability and validity of key-feature cases for the self-assessment of colon and rectal surgeons. Ann Surg. 2008;248(2):252–8.
21. Zamani S, Amini M, Masoumi SZ, Delavari S, Namaki MJ, Kojuri J. The comparison of the key feature of clinical reasoning and multiple choice examinations in clinical decision makings ability. Biomed Res [Internet]. 2017 [cited 2021 Nov 26];28(3):1115–9. Available from: http://apps.webofknowledge.com/InboundService.do?Func=Frame&product=WOS&action=retrieve&SrcApp=EndNote&Init=Yes&SrcAuth=ResearchSoft&mode=FullRecord&UT=000396822900024
22. Downing S. What is good item discrimination? In: Yudkowsky SMD& R, editor. Assessment in Health Professions Education. New York: Routledge; 2009. p. 108.
23. Nikendei C, Mennin S, Weyrich P, Kraus B, Zipfel S, Schrauth M, et al. Effects of a supplementary final year curriculum on students' clinical reasoning skills as assessed by key-feature examination. Med Teach. 2009;31(9):438–42.
24. Rademakers J, ten Cate T, Bar P. Progress testing with short answer questions. Med Teach. 2005;27(7):578–82.
25. Bland JM, Altman DG. Statistics notes: Cronbach's alpha. BMJ. 1997;
26. Bordage G, Carretier H, Bertrand R, Page G. Comparing times and performances of french and english - Speaking candidates taking a national examination of clinical decision - Making skills. Acad Med [Internet]. 1995 May 1 [cited 2021 Nov 27];70(5):359–65. Available from: https://europepmc.org/article/med/7748379

27. Eva KW, Wood TJ, Riddle J, Touchie C, Bordage G. How clinical features are presented matters to weaker diagnosticians: Language matters. Med Educ [Internet]. 2010 Aug 1 [cited 2021 Nov 27];44(8):775–85. Available from: https://onlinelibrary.wiley.com/doi/full/10.1111/j.1365-2923.2010.03705.x
28. Norman G, Bordage G, Page G, Keane D. How specific is case specificity? Med Educ [Internet]. 2006 Jul 1 [cited 2021 Nov 27];40(7):618–23. Available from: https://onlinelibrary.wiley.com/doi/full/10.1111/j.1365-2929.2006.02511.x
29. Wass V, Van Der Vleuten C, Shatzer J, Jones R. Assessment of clinical competence. Vol. 357, Lancet. Elsevier; 2001. p. 945–9.
30. Tamblyn R, Abrahamowicz M, Dauphinee D, Wenghofer E, Jacques A, Klass D, et al. Physician scores on a national clinical skills examination as predictors of complaints to medical regulatory authorities. J Am Med Assoc [Internet]. 2007 Sep 5 [cited 2021 Nov 26];298(9):993–1001. Available from: https://jamanetwork.com/journals/jama/fullarticle/208633
31. Tamblyn R, Abrahamowicz M, Dauphinee D, Wenghofer E, Jacques A, Klass D, et al. Influence of physicians' management and communication ability on patients' persistence with antihypertensive medication. Arch Intern Med [Internet]. 2010 Jun 28 [cited 2021 Nov 26];170(12):1064–72. Available from: https://jamanetwork.com/journals/jamainternalmedicine/fullarticle/416089
32. Korenstein D, Thomas D, Foldes C, Ross J, Halm E, McGinn T. An evidence-based domestic violence education programme for internal medicine residents. Teach Learn Med. 2003;15(4):262–6.
33. Doucet M, Purdy R, Kaufman D, Langille D. Comparison of problem-based learning and lecture format in continuing medical education on headache diagnosis and management. Med Educ. 1998;32(6):590–6.
34. Eva K, Wood T. Can the strength of candidates be discriminated based on ability to circumvent the biasing effect of prose? Acad Med. 2003;78(10 Supplement):78–81.
35. Schuwirth L, Gorter S, van der Heijde D, Rethans J, Brauer J, Houben H, et al. The role of a computerised case-based testing procedure in practice performance assessment. Adv Heal Sci Educ Theory Pr. 2005;10(2):145–55.
36. Schuwirth LWT, Verheggen MM, Van Der Vleuten CPM, Boshuizen HPA, Dinant GJ. Do short cases elicit different thinking processes than factual knowledge questions do? Med Educ [Internet]. 2001 Apr 22 [cited 2021 Nov 27];35(4):348–56. Available from: https://onlinelibrary.wiley.com/doi/full/10.1046/j.1365-2923.2001.00771.x

# Chapter 6
# A-Type MCQs

**Hosam Eldeen Elsadig Gasmalla**
**and Mohamed Elnajid Mustafa Mohamed Tahir**

**Abstract** In this chapter, the authors focus on the construction of A-type MCQs that go beyond merely assessing recall, into assessing high levels of the cognitive domain, and examples are utilized extensively.

*By the end of this chapter, the reader is expected to be able to*

1. Describe the structure of A-type MCQs.
2. Detect the common mistakes in writing MCQs.
3. Construct A-type MCQs for assessment of high cognitive level.

**Keywords** A-type MCQs · Restricted response items

Test item writing may be as much art as science. –Steven M. Downing

## Background

As mentioned in Chap. 2, the commonly used multiple-choice questions include true or false questions (X-type), single best or single correct answer (A-type), and extended matching questions (R-type). Other newer formats of multiple-choice questions include key feature items and script concordance items.

A-type MCQ is a variety of multiple-choice questions. It was first introduced by Frederick J. Kellyjn in 1914 [1, 2], and it has been used since the 1950s in medical schools [3]. Moreover, it is the most used assessment tool in medical education [4].

H. E. E. Gasmalla (✉)
University of Warwick, Coventry, United Kingdom

Al Neelain University, Khartoum, Sudan
e-mail: hosam.mohammed@warwick.ac.uk

M. E. M. Mohamed Tahir
Physiologist at the Faculty of Medicine, University of Medical Science and Technology, Khartoum, Sudan

Nile University, Khartoum, Sudan



H. E. E. Gasmalla et al. (eds.), *Written Assessment in Medical Education*,
https://doi.org/10.1007/978-3-031-11752-7_6

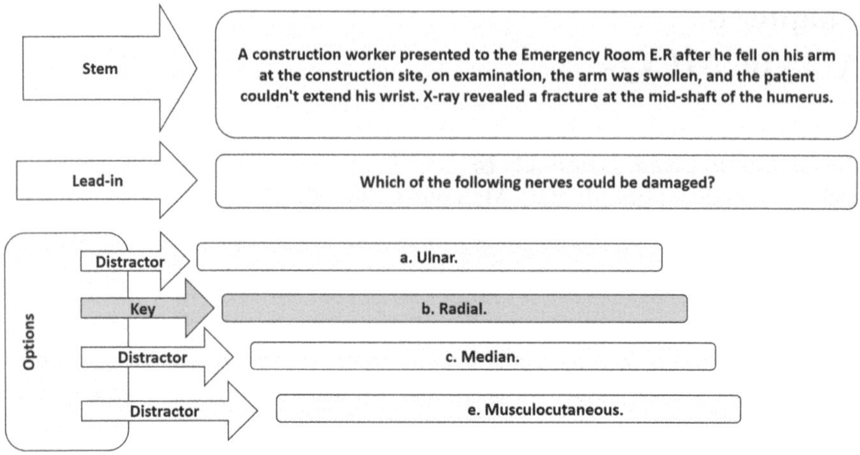


**Fig. 6.1** Structure of A-type MCQs

It is an objective assessment tool with a restricted response. It consists of a stem (which could be a scenario or a clinical vignette), lead-in question, and options. The options vary between three and five (usually three to four distractors and a correct answer, the key), as in Fig. 6.1 [5, 6].

There are two varieties for A-type MCQs: contextual and noncontextual.

## *Contextual Items*

A contextual (scenario-based or vignette-rich) item contains a rich scenario in the "stem"; they can assess higher levels of the cognitive domain [7]. *An example of a contextual item is given below*:

**Stem**
A 35 year-old-woman presented to the ER with severe abdominal pain. History revealed that the pain is constant, recurrent, and related to fatty meals. Cholecystitis was suspected as a provisional diagnosis. Ultrasonography was requested.

**Lead-in**
During ultrasonography, what is the most important abdominal region the doctor should focus on?

**Options**
(a) Epigastric.
(b) Left lumbar.
(c) Left iliac fossa.
(d) Right hypochondrium.*

## *Noncontextual Items*

Unlike the contextual items, the noncontextual items come without scenario; thus, it is limited to the lower levels of the cognitive domain. *An example of noncontextual is given below*:

**Lead-in**
In which of the following abdominal regions the gallbladder is located?

**Options**
(a) Epigastric.
(b) Left lumbar.
(c) Right iliac fossa.
(d) Right hypochondrium.*

## *Advantages and Limitations*

**Advantages**

*Objective*: Marking A-type MCQs is not subjective, recently, computer-based MCQs can perform marking and analysis of test results without human intervention.

*Validity and reliability*: Test results of a well developed A-type MCQs are reliable, and this format presents evidence of validity. Since many items can be introduced in one test, this provides optimal coverage of learning outcomes and makes fulfilling the blueprint easier. The objectivity of marking and the ability to assess variable cognitive domains add to the validity and reliability.

*Feasible*: It can be used to assess a large amount of knowledge in a relatively short duration. It can also be introduced to a large number of candidates at once.

**Limitations**

As a written assessment tool, A-type MCQs can only assess the cognitive domain. Well-constructed MCQs demand time and great effort and the construction depends on the capability of the writer. Since the number of options is limited to not more than five (sometimes four), thus, it is prone to guessing, the assessor cannot tell if the candidate has answered the question because he or she knows the answer, or it was just guessing. Even though the candidate has selected the correct answer, it does not show the explanation of how he or she has figured it out.

**Practical Application***When to use A-type MCQs?*

A-type MCQs are used to assess competencies at all levels of the cognitive domain.

*When not to use A-type MCQs?*

Not to be used when assessing competencies related to psychomotor and affective domains, as well as any form of expanded elaboration such as reflections

## How to Construct A-Type MCQs?

Preparing an A-type MCQ is a matter of finesse; it is important to consider the qualities of the stem, lead-in, and options.

### *Stem*

It is a given scenario that contains relevant facts and information. The purpose of the stem is to present a scenario to challenge/assess clinical reasoning/higher cognitive functions. When writing the stem, consider the following:

- *Contents*: The stem can contain an image, audio, or video.
- *Relevance*: No need to write or include anything that is irrelevant.
- *Language*: The used language should be clear and simple, considering that the candidates might not be native speakers.
- *Grammar*: The scenario is a storytelling section; consider the consistency when using past and/or present tenses.
- *Abbreviations*: Avoid abbreviations, instead, write the full term in the stem.
- *Age*: Write it with hyphens as "five-year-old/5-year-old" if it is a substitute for a noun or if it proceeds the noun (e.g., a five-year-old patient is brought to the hospital). Age can be written without hyphens if the noun comes before it "my son has just turned five years old." Note that in this example the word "years" is plural, unlike the first example.

**Practical Applications***Useful templates*: **Refer to the following templates when writing the stem.**

*Template one*: A (patient information, such as age and gender) complains of (symptoms). On examination (signs). What is the possible diagnosis (options: list of diagnoses)? Or, which one of the following muscles could be affected (options: list of muscles)? Or absence/or deficiency of which one of the following enzymes can explain this condition? (Options: list of enzymes).

*Template two*: A (patient information, such as age and gender) is brought to the emergency room following (event such road traffic accident), he/she is (symptoms). On examination (signs). Investigations show (lab. results). Which one of the following nerves could be injured (options: list of nerves)?

*Template three*: (duration) after (event such as eating a meal), a (patient information, such as age and gender) complains of (symptoms). Investigations show (lab. results) which one of the following (organisms) is most likely to be the cause of this condition? (Options: list of nerves).

## *Lead-in*

It is a statement that usually comes in the form of a question. When writing the lead-in, consider the following:

- *Constructive alignment*: It should be consistent with the learning outcomes; each lead-in has to test one specific learning outcome or to address one specific problem.
- *Clarity*: It has to be specific, clear, and in the form of a question that ends with a question mark. The question itself can be answered without reading the options.
- *Simplicity*: Avoid using negative construction of the sentence by using words such as "EXCEPT" or "NOT." It creates irrelevant difficulties.

## *Options*

The options are (*distractors*) plus one option which is the answer (*key*). During writing the options, make sure that your writing is of high quality, to achieve that, consider the following:

- *Homogeneity*: All options must be homogenous, i.e., all are diagnoses, lab results, signs, symptoms, and lengths.
- *Length*: Options are better to be short if possible, with the same length.
- *Arrangement*: They should be arranged in a logical manner (numerical, alphabetical, or sequential).
- *Key answer*: During writing the one correct answer, the *Key*, it is advisable to avoid making it obvious or debatable.

## *Distractors*

All the options (except for one) comprises wrong answers, their function is to distract the candidate from the correct answer, that is why they are known as *distractors*, write them to be:

- Based on common student errors, misconceptions, and misunderstandings.
- Adequately different from the answer "*Key*" (for those who have learned the objectives of the course).
- Distracting only those students who have not mastered or learned the objectives of the course.

*The functionality of distractors*: Distractor that gains responses less than 5% of the total responses to the item is considered as nonfunctional.

## What Is the Optimal Number of Options in an Item: Five, Four, or Three?

It is important to mention that in this book, and while we are adopting the four-options approach, we do not necessarily promote it. There is evidence in the published literature that support five, four, or even three options in the item. In this section, we present to you all the evidence along with the argument associated with each approach.

Constructing five options is considered convenient although it is arbitrary [3]. In terms of the functionality of distractors, increasing the number of distractors does not necessarily mean that all of them are functional [8].

### What Is the Justification for Reducing the Number of Options?

The inclination to reduce the number of options per item comes from the fact that there are many nonfunctioning distractors (NFDs) [8]. Many authors recommend using four options (or even three) instead of five [9–12]. However, there are many issues to be discussed and considered. Below is a summary of an argument of those who oppose reducing the number of options:

### Is Reducing the Number of Options Is the Only Way to Minimize NFDs?

Developing items with functioning distractors is a solution too; it requires training the test developers, and development processes and methods to ensure distractors' efficacy. In this case, there will be no need to decrease the number of options.

Reducing the number of options increases the odds of guessing the correct answer.

### Decreasing the Options from Five to Four Has Undesirable Effects

A meta-analysis conducted by [10] concluded that reducing the number of options from five to four has led to a reduction in the discrimination index by 0.04 (the questions became less discriminative), and the reliability was also decreased by 0.035. However, this meta-analysis concluded that three options per item are acceptable.

### Evidence Evaluation: Are Studies that Prefer Four Options Credible?

Most of the studies that prefer four options are based on items developed in local medical schools, and not on items develop by credentialing bodies, in which the item undergoes rigorous revision before it is published. Other studies are from school education or another nonmedical education context, which must be considered in evaluating the evidence.

Can we Revisit the Definition of NFDs?

Item difficulty affects the definition of NFDs. The current definition of distractors efficacy does not consider the effect of item difficulty. A new way to calculate item difficulty was proposed by [8], in which the effect of item difficulty is considered. Applying this formula (or any other proposed definition of distractors efficacy that considers the effect of item difficulty) on the previously published work may change their recommendations of adopting four options.

## Item Flaws (Table 6.1)

### *Examples of Item Flaws: General Flaws*

The following are examples of item flaws [13–15], each one is provided by an explanation for the flaw and how to reconstruct the question; the key answer in each question is indicated by (*) (Table 6.2).

### *Examples of Item Flaws: Flaws Contribute to Irrelevant Difficulty (Table 6.3)*

## Constructing High Cognitive Level A-Type MCQs

**Table 6.1** Categories of item flaws

| General flaws | Flaws contribute to irrelevant difficulty |
|---|---|
| Grammatical mistakes | Poorly arranged numeric data |
| Very long correct answer | Negatively constructed items |
| Repeated word in the stem and options | Using phrases like "none of the above" or "all of the above" |
| Merging more than one item in one answer | Unclear or vague lead-in or options |
| Long and exhausting options | The question cannot be answered by covering the options "hand-cover test" (in contextual MCQs) |
| Using absolute terms | |
| Using nonlogical option | |
| Using irrelevant (nonhomogeneous) options | |

**Table 6.2** Examples of item flaws: general flaws

| Flaw category | Example | Reconstruction/comment |
|---|---|---|
| Grammatical mistakes | Which one of the following are part of the reflex that responds to an increase in arterial pressure?<br>(a) The decreased firing of the baroreceptors.<br>(b) Stimulated sympathetic activity to the ventricle.<br>(c) Stimulated parasympathetic activity to the SA node.*<br>(d) Increased parasympathetic stimulation to the ventricles. | Which one of the following is part of the reflex that responds to an increase in arterial pressure?<br>(a) The decreased firing of the baroreceptors.<br>(b) Stimulated sympathetic activity to the ventricle.<br>(c) Stimulated parasympathetic activity to the SA node.*<br>(d) Increased parasympathetic stimulation to the ventricles.<br>In the stem, the word "are" indicates faulty grammar, and using the word "respond" is incorrect, the correct word is "response."<br>The question itself cannot be answered using hand-cover. |
| | Which one of the following branches of the aorta are responsible for the blood supply of the cecum?<br>(a) Renal.<br>(b) Celiac.<br>(c) Median sacral.<br>(d) Superior mesenteric.*<br>The target answer is one artery, thus putting the word "are" in the lead-in confuses the student and sends the wrong message about the integrity of the exam. | Which one of the following branches of the aorta is responsible for the blood supply of the cecum?<br>(a) Renal.<br>(b) Celiac.<br>(c) Median sacral.<br>(d) Superior mesenteric.*<br>Now the grammar is consistent, and the purpose of the question is clear. |
| Very long correct answer | Iron is:<br>(a) Mainly stored in the form of hemosiderin.<br>(b) The requirement is greater in males.<br>(c) Absorption is greater in anemic patients. than normal subject*<br>(d) Mainly stored in the spleen | This item has many mistakes in it; first, it is not in a form of a question; second, it cannot pass the hand-cover test, which makes it unclear. And of course, the answer is different from the distractors in being distinguishably long.<br>Such questions are difficult to be reconstructed. |
| | Located within the cubital fossa is the ____ nerve:<br>(a) Ulnar.<br>(b) Axillary.<br>(c) Lateral pectoral.<br>(d) Median nerve with the artery lateral to it.*<br>An effort has been put to make (e) a correct answer; the student can notice that easily | Which one of the following is located within the cubital fossa?<br>(a) Ulnar.<br>(b) Median.*<br>(c) Axillary.<br>(d) Lateral pectoral.<br>Converted into questions format rather than fill in the space<br>Note that the "Median nerve" has been moved after reconstruction from (e) to (b) to maintain the arrangement of the options according to their length. |

(continued)

**Table 6.2** (continued)

| Flaw category | Example | Reconstruction/comment |
|---|---|---|
| Repeated word in the stem and options | What is the muscle that originates from the subscapular fossa?<br>(a) Subscapularis.*<br>(b) Supraspinatus.<br>(c) Latissimus dorsi.<br>(d) Pectoralis major.<br>Obviously, the answer is subscapularis! | Which one of the following is the muscle that originates from the anterior surface of the scapula?<br>(a) Subscapularis.*<br>(b) Supraspinatus.<br>(c) Latissimus dorsi.<br>(d) Pectoralis major.<br>"Subscapular fossa" has been replaced by "anterior surface of the scapula," with the same meaning. |
| | The osmotic water ($H_2O$) movement across a semi-permeable membrane is defined as:<br>(a) Active transport.<br>(b) Diffusion.<br>(c) Osmosis.*<br>(d) Tonicity. | Which of the following terms is best defined "The passage of water ($H_2O$) across a semi-permeable membrane"?<br>(a) Active transport.<br>(b) Diffusion.<br>(c) Osmosis.*<br>(d) Tonicity. |
| Merging more than one item in one answer | Regarding heart failure, raised JVP could be found in:<br>(a) Right-sided heart failure.*<br>(b) Congestive heart failure.<br>(c) Left-sided heart failure.<br>(d) a and b are correct. | In this question, the correct answer is also part of another distractor (Congestive heart failure) and this merging is in (d). merging can reduce the actual number of functioning distractors, in this case, there are only three (a, b, and c) |
| | The main motor innervation of the diaphragm is achieved by:<br>(a) C3.<br>(b) C4.<br>(c) C5.<br>(d) C3 and C4.<br>The diaphragm is innervated mainly from C4, with contributions from C3 and C5; (b), (d), and (e) are all part of the correct answer, so what is the correct answer exactly? How confusing is this question? To edit this question correctly, each item of the distractors must be written with its own identity, "i.e., it must be independent and not be part of any other item in the distractors". | The main motor innervation of the diaphragm is achieved by:<br>(a) C3.<br>(b) C4.*<br>(c) C5.<br>(d) C6.<br>OR: Motor innervation of the diaphragm is achieved by which one of the following?<br>(a) C1 and C2.<br>(b) C3, 4, and 5.*<br>(c) C6, 7, and 8.<br>(d) T1 and T2<br>Each item now is independent. |

(continued)

**Table 6.2** (continued)

| Flaw category | Example | Reconstruction/comment |
|---|---|---|
| Long and exhausting options | A 60-year-old male patient was brought to the Emergency Department in a deep coma. When history was taken from his daughter, she stated that he complained of a very severe headache immediately before passing into a coma. According to her, he described the headache as the worst headache of his life. Bearing in mind the most likely diagnosis, which of the following statements is correct?<br>(a) The cause of coma in this patient is the increase in the intracranial pressure (ICP) which jeopardized the cerebral perfusion pressure (CPP).*<br>(b) The risk of the sudden death of patients with this diagnosis at the time of initial presentation is not high.<br>(c) The description of the headache given in the scenario is not of significant value in suspecting the diagnosis.<br>(d) The diagnosis of this condition is based exclusively on the history and neurological examination. | This question is in form of true/false items rather than A-type MCQ.<br>The lead-in and the options are too long, after reading each option the student may forget what the main question at the lead-in was. |
| | Drinking 1 liter of pure water is expected to:<br>(a) Induce a greater increase in the volume of extracellular fluid than intracellular fluid.<br>(b) Induce a greater decrease in osmolarity of extracellular fluid than intracellular fluid.<br>(c) Induce a greater increase in the volume of plasma than interstitial fluid.<br>(d) Induce a greater decrease in osmolarity of plasma than interstitial fluid.<br>The allotted duration for each question in the exam will be very short considering this one, besides the long options contributing to the irrelevant complexity. | This question does not assess a specific idea; instead, it generalizes the lead-in question.<br>To make it right, one can choose from the several ideas included in the question and turn it into MCQ, note that all reconstructions should of course follow the objectives in their arrangement in the blueprint.<br>Another form of long and exhausting options: repeating words in all options. |

(continued)

**Table 6.2** (continued)

| Flaw category | Example | Reconstruction/comment |
|---|---|---|
| Using absolute or vague terms | Babinski s sign:<br>(a) Always a lower motor neuron lesions sign.<br>(b) Characterized downward of the big toe.<br>(c) Usually, it goes with upper motor neuron lesions signs.*<br>(d) Can be seen in a normal awake adult. | This item has many mistakes in it; first, it is not in a form of a question; second, using vague words like "always," "can be," and "usually." Third, it cannot pass the hand-cover test, which makes it more ambiguous. |
| | The parasympathetic innervation of the heart:<br>(a) Is derived from the vagi.*<br>(b) Increases the heart rate.<br>(c) Increases force of contraction.<br>(d) Increases the blood flow in coronary arteries.<br>The word "always" is absolute; it gives a hint to the student either to exclude this option or to consider it an answer. | After removing the word "always," the rest is the same.<br>Examples of absolute or vague words: always, usually, sometimes, never, generally, commonly, almost, can be, could be, maybe, and might be. |
| Using nonlogical option | Which of the following hormones is secreted by the kidney?<br>(a) Growth hormone.<br>(b) Thyroid hormone.<br>(c) Erythropoietin.*<br>(d) Nephron.<br>The nephron is not a hormone, which excludes one of the options from the list automatically. | Which one of the following hormones is secreted by the kidney and affects hematopoiesis?<br>(a) Growth hormone.<br>(b) Thyroid hormone.<br>(c) Erythropoietin.*<br>(d) Prolactin.<br>All the options are fulfilling the same category: hormones. The question can be answered by hand-covering the options. |
| | Which one of the following joints is synovial?<br>(a) Humerus.<br>(b) Hip joint.*<br>(c) Coronal suture.<br>(d) Symphysis pubis.<br>The humerus is not a joint, which excludes one of the options from the list automatically. | Which one of the following joints is synovial?<br>(a) Hip joint.*<br>(b) Costochondral.<br>(c) Coronal suture.<br>(d) Symphysis pubis.<br>Now all of them are fulfilling the same category: joints. However, it is still not preferred as it does not fulfill cover the options rule. |

(continued)

**Table 6.2** (continued)

| Flaw category | Example | Reconstruction/comment |
|---|---|---|
| Using irrelevant (nonhomogeneous) options | A good location for pulse examination of the radial artery is:<br>(a) At the wrist.*<br>(b) Side of the neck.<br>(c) Femoral triangle.<br>(d) Dorsum of the foot.<br>All the options (except for the wrist) are in the same category (lower limb locations); the radial artery is in the upper limb, which makes it easy to be sorted as an answer. | In which of the following locations the radial artery is best palpated?<br>(a) Wrist.*<br>(b) Cubital fossa.<br>(c) Axilla.<br>(d) Dorsum of the hand.<br>All options are homogenous; the stem is in the form of a question and the item can be answered even with the options covered. |
| | The nerve that is responsible for the extension at the wrist joint is:<br>(a) Ulnar nerve.<br>(b) Radial nerve.*<br>(c) Median nerve.<br>(d) Femoral nerve.<br>Although all the options here are in the same category (all are nerves), the femoral nerve is not among the nerves of the upper limb, which makes it easy to exclude (Compare this with the example in "7"). | Which one of the following nerves is responsible for the extension at the wrist joint?<br>(a) Ulnar.<br>(b) Radial.*<br>(c) Median nerve.<br>(d) Axillary nerve.<br>The femoral nerve is simply replaced by the axillary nerve, a nerve in the upper limb; making the distractors homogeneous is a fair way to increase the difficulty of the question and yet keep it flawless.<br>Note that the stem has been reshaped in a form of a question. |

There are many levels for each learning domain according to bloom taxonomy, the cognitive domain levels are as follows:

1. Remember (Knowledge)
2. Understand (Comprehension)
3. Apply (Application)
4. Analyze (Analysis)
5. Evaluate (Evaluation)
6. Create (Synthesis)

In this section, we used examples of Human Anatomy questions, the general belief is that "Gross Anatomy" is all about "recalling" facts only, we are challenging this by bringing the following examples in all levels of the cognitive domain.

1. *Remember (Knowledge)*: the ability to recall facts.

   *Example*: What is the name of the most Suitable abdominal incision for appendectomy?

   (a) Kocher.
   (b) Midline.

**Table 6.3** Examples of item flaws: flaws contribute to the irrelevant difficulty

| Flaw category | Example | Reconstruction and comment |
|---|---|---|
| Poorly arranged numeric data | The total body water in a 70 kg adult male is about:<br>(a) 40 liters*<br>(b) 60 liters<br>(c) 25 liters<br>(d) 28 liters<br>The answer although is clear for a medical student, this bad arrangement of numbers makes it difficult. | What is the amount of total body water (in liters) in a 70 kg adult male?<br>(a) 60<br>(b) 40<br>(c) 28<br>(d) 25<br>This arrangement makes it easier. Note that the stem has also been changed into a form of a question, which resulted in removing the repeated word (liter) from the options. |
| | The sternal angle (angle of Louis) is located at the level of the lower border of the following thoracic vertebra:<br>(a) 2nd.<br>(b) 3rd.<br>(c) 5th.<br>(d) 4th.*<br>The answer although is clear for a medical student, this bad arrangement of numbers makes it difficult. | With relation to the vertebrae, at which level is the sternal angle (angle of Louis) located?<br>(a) 2nd.<br>(b) 3rd.<br>(c) 4th.*<br>(d) 5th.<br>This arrangement makes it easier. Note that the stem has been reshaped in a form of a question. |
| Negatively constructed items | One of the following is NOT true about ammonium production:<br>(a) It is mainly a function of PCT.*<br>(b) The source is mainly glutamine.<br>(c) It is a low-capacity high gradient system.<br>(d) It is increased when the urine pH is low. | Negatively constructed items are usually difficult to be reconstructed. In this case, it is recommended to delete such questions |
| | All of the following can cause hyperkinesia EXCEPT:<br>(a) Lesion of the caudate nucleus.<br>(b) Lesion of the subthalamic nucleus.<br>(c) Lesion of substantia nigra.*<br>Lesion of putamen nucleus. | |

(continued)

**Table 6.3** (continued)

| Flaw category | Example | Reconstruction and comment |
|---|---|---|
| Using phrases like "none of the above" or "all of the above" | Coughing of blood is known as:<br>(a) Hemodialysis.<br>(b) Hematemesis.<br>(c) Epistaxis.<br>(d) None of the above.* | This question has many mistakes in it; first, the options are *nonhomogeneous* and *nonlogical*; second, the selected answer has no relation with the question.<br>Such questions are difficult to be reconstructed. |
| | Regarding chest pain:<br>(a) It could be of cardiac or pulmonary origin.<br>(b) Cardiac pain is relieved by rest.<br>(c) Pulmonary pain is aggravated by coughing & deep breathing.<br>(d) All the above statements are correct.* | This item has many mistakes in it; first, it is not in a form of a question; second, it cannot pass the hand-cover test, which makes it unclear.<br>And of course, the answer is different from the distractors in being distinguishably long.<br>Such questions are difficult to be reconstructed. |

(c) Pfannenstiel.
(d) McBurney's.*

2. *Understand (Comprehension)*: the ability to digest and understand gained knowledge.

   *Example*: A resident doctor in the emergency medicine department has been called to examine an old patient in the ward of the cardiology, the patient was severely ill, with marked weight loss, on examination pulse rate was 100 bpm, respiratory rate 22 per minute, neck veins were engorged, heart sounds were diminished, and the liver was enlarged (hepatomegaly).

   The nurse mentioned to the doctor that the patient has been admitted a few days ago and was diagnosed as having myocardial infarction; she also mentioned that he is under chemotherapy.

   The history and the signs were strongly suggestive of "cardiac tamponade."

   The neck veins were engorged due to the congestion in which vein?

   (a) Azygos vein.
   (b) Hemiazygos.
   (c) Left subclavian.
   (d) Superior vena cava.*

   *Explanation*: To answer this question, the student has to "*explain*" the reason for the engorged neck veins by determining the site of congestion according to his knowledge "*recall*" of anatomy.

3. *Apply (Application of knowledge)*: the ability to use knowledge.

   *Example*: A right-handed patient is having difficulty in opening a plastic cork of Coca-Cola bottle, what is the affected muscle?

   (a) Brachialis.
   (b) Biceps brachii.*
   (c) Brachioradialis.
   (d) Coracobrachialis.

   *Explanation*: Background information regarding the origin and insertion of muscles are "*used*" to determine the resulting action. The student has to apply the factual knowledge.

4. *Analyze (Analysis)*: the ability to defragment concepts into their basic parts and to identify the relation between them.

   *Example*: Kamal is a 65-year-old accountant brought to the E.R complaining of severe and sharp chest pain, he told the resident doctor that the pain was initially in his shoulder, he is a known diabetic, hypertensive and heavy smoker for 10 years.

   ECG showed ST-segment elevation in V1, V2, and V3. Following workup, the doctor made the diagnosis of myocardial infarction.

   Which coronary artery could be affected?

   (a) Circumflex.
   (b) Left marginal.
   (c) Right marginal.
   (d) Anterior interventricular.*

   *Explanation*: *Breaking down* the ECG readings to indicate the site of infarction and *relating* this to the blood supply of that site lead the student to the answer.

5. *Evaluation*: The ability to conclude results or to reach a judgment or diagnosis.

   *Used expressions*: choose, conclude, decide, determine, evaluate, judge, agree, interpret, and estimate.

   *Example (1)*: Khalid is a candidate for AV fistula in preparation for renal dialysis, the doctor performed the modified Allen's test for the patient, when the doctor released the pressure from the ulnar artery the hand did not flush completely; he considered it as "negative modified Allen's test."

   What is the artery that should be avoided when performing the AV fistula?

   (a) Ulnar artery.
   (b) Radial artery.
   (c) Brachial artery.

(d) Anterior interosseous artery.

*Example (2)*:

*This question is testing simple recall*:

*First question*: What is the suitable abdominal incision for an appendectomy?

(a) Midline incision.
(b) Subcostal (Kocher) incision.
(c) Suprapubic (Pfannenstiel) incision.
(d) Muscle splitting (McBurney's) incision.*

*Now, this is how to test evaluation*:

*Second (modified) question*: Huda is a 22-year-old university student, who presented to E.R. with severe abdominal pain that started in the center of the abdomen before it became localized to the right iliac fossa. She was complaining of nausea and vomiting.

O/E she was ill, laying with the right hip flexed; when asked to describe the location of the pain, she pointed at the right iliac fossa; the doctor detected pain in that area among palpation of the left iliac fossa.

After investigations, the doctor made the diagnosis and took her to the operation room. Choose a suitable abdominal incision for this patient?

(a) Kocher.
(b) Midline.
(c) Pfannenstiel.
(d) McBurney's.*

*Explanation*: The *first question* is directly about the suitable abdominal incision, the diagnosis is already mentioned; in the *Second (modified) question*, the diagnosis is removed so that the main concern of the question is to reach the *diagnosis (Evaluation)*; to do this, the student has to use the given anatomical facts (*recall*) and correlate them (referred pain, fixed flexed hip), which is (*comprehension*) and (*application*), and the student also has to *analyze* facts (pain in the right iliac fossa among palpation of the left iliac fossa: explanation: peritoneal fluids movements).

Note that the diagnosis of appendicitis is mostly based on anatomical facts.

**Take-Home Message**

A-type MCQs are a variety of multiple-choice questions. It is a tool to assess competencies related to the cognitive domain (except "creating"). It consists of a stem, a lead-in question, and options. The options vary between three and five (usually three to four distractors and a correct answer, the key).

Constructing A-type MCQs is a matter of finesse; poorly constructed items can diminish the degree of validity of the interpretation of test scores.

## References


1. Madaus GF, O'Dwyer LM. A short history of performance assessment: Lessons learned. Phi Delta Kappan.. 1999;80(9):688.
2. Liu OL, Lee H-S, Linn MC. An investigation of explanation multiple-choice items in science assessment. Educational Assessment.. 2011;16(3):164–84.
3. Anderson J. For multiple choice questions. Medical teacher.. 1979;1(1):37–42.
4. Wadi MM, Nour-El-Din M, Qureshi M-G. Writing MCQ in a reverse way: feasibility and usability. Education in Medicine Journal. 2017;9(3).
5. Case SM, Swanson DB. Constructing written test questions for the basic and clinical sciences. 3 ed: National Board of Medical Examiners Philadelphia; 2000.
6. Wojtczak A. Glossary of medical education terms: AMEE; 2003.
7. Case SM, Swanson DB. Constructing written test questions for the basic and clinical sciences: National Board of Medical Examiners Philadelphia; 1998.
8. Raymond MR, Stevens C, Bucak SD. The optimal number of options for multiple-choice questions on high-stakes tests: application of a revised index for detecting nonfunctional distractors. Advances in Health Sciences Education. 2019;24(1):141–50.
9. Vyas R, Supe A. Multiple choice questions: a literature review on the optimal number of options. Natl Med J India. 2008;21(3):130–3.
10. Rodriguez MC. Three options are optimal for multiple-choice items: A meta-analysis of 80 years of research. Educational measurement: issues and practice. 2005;24(2):3–13.
11. Tarrant M, Ware J, Mohammed AM. An assessment of functioning and non-functioning distractors in multiple-choice questions: a descriptive analysis. BMC medical education. 2009; 9(1):1–8.
12. Kilgour JM, Tayyaba S. An investigation into the optimal number of distractors in single-best answer exams. Advances in Health Sciences Education. 2016;21(3):571–85.
13. Al-Wardy NM. Assessment methods in undergraduate medical education. Sultan Qaboos Univ Med J. 2010;10(2):203–9.
14. Abdalla ME, Gaffar AM, Suliman RA. Constructing A-Type Multiple Choice Questions (MCQs): Step By Step Manual: Abdelrahim Mutwakel Gaffar; 2011.
15. Touchie L. Guidelines for the development of multiple-choice questions. Medical Council of Canada. 2010.

# Chapter 7
# R-Type MCQs (Extended Matching Questions)

**Hosam Eldeen Elsadig Gasmalla**
**and Mohamed Elnajid Mustafa Mohamed Tahir**

**Abstract** R-type questions (or extended matching questions) are a type of MCQs that are rich in context. They are organized into options and stem questions led by a lead-in; the candidate must match the stems with the provided options. The options, stem questions, and lead-in collectively make one item that addresses one theme. R-type items are objective. They can assess clinical reasoning. Improving the psychometric properties depends on the number of options as well as the stems, increasing the number of options will enhance the discrimination index and reduce the guessing probability of the items, yet it will increase the time required for the test. Thus 8 options are recommended to get the ultimate use of time, discrimination, and difficulty indices; increasing the number of items up to 100 will ensure reliability.

*By the end of this chapter, the reader is expected to be able to*

1. Describe the structure of R-type MCQs.
2. Construct quality R-type MCQs.
3. Pinpoint the psychometric properties of R-type MCQs.

**Keywords** R-type MCQs · Restricted response items

H. E. E. Gasmalla (✉)
University of Warwick, Coventry, United Kingdom

Al Neelain University, Khartoum, Sudan
e-mail: hosam.mohammed@warwick.ac.uk

M. E. M. Mohamed Tahir
Physiologist at the Faculty of Medicine, University of Medical Science and Technology, Khartoum, Sudan

Nile University, Khartoum, Sudan



H. E. Gasmalla et al. (eds.), *Written Assessment in Medical Education*,
https://doi.org/10.1007/978-3-031-11752-7_7

## Introduction

Clinical reasoning can be described as the cognitive processes by which the doctor can reach the most probable diagnosis of the patient and put a plan of management [1, 2]. The assessment of clinical reasoning is the core of the assessment in medical education, and the quest is always about developing a better assessment tool that is reliable and feasible.

R-type multiple-choice questions (also known as extended matching questions) were introduced in the 1990s as an additional form of MCQs. Although A-type MCQs can be introduced to a large number of students at a time, their scoring is objective, easy, and score's interpretations are considered reliable, but doubts were raised about the ability of A-type to assess the application of knowledge and clinical reasoning [3, 4], besides the concerns of the chance of correct guessing [5]. Concerns about the number of options for each question have always been there. The debate of increasing the number of options takes into consideration that the introduction of a large number of options per item will mimic the situation in clinical scenarios; in addition, in the same assessment there is no need to make the same number of options for each question for the number of options is different according to the content of the question. Thus, the variation in the number of options within the same assessment creates flexibility that makes assessment construction easier [6].

On the other hand, constructed-response (or open-ended) questions can assess the higher levels of cognitive functions and clinical reasoning, but their narrow coverage of the contents makes the interpretations driven from scores less valid. The ambiguity of the intended answer of the student and/or the intentions of the examiner reduces the reliability and imposes logistic difficulties due to the scoring process and its subjectivity [7].

Thus, R-type MCQs come at midway between both A-type MCQs and constructed-response questions: a large number of options reduce the chance of correct guessing and allow for assessment of higher levels of cognitive domain as well as clinical reasoning, thus overcoming the disadvantages of A-type MCQs. In addition, the objectivity of R-type in scoring overcomes the disadvantages of free-response (or open-ended) questions, and scoring itself is easy. Furthermore, many other assessment tools were considered for the assessment of clinical reasoning, such as script concordance tests. However, the script concordance test is mainly used for postgraduate candidates, and it is laborious to score, in addition to that its suitability to be constructed as a computer-based assessment is complex. This makes extended matching questions one of the best assessment tools recommended for computer-based assessment [1, 8].

There is a movement toward R-type questions since the 2000s. In the UK, it has been introduced in the examinations of the Royal College of Obstetricians and Gynaecologists since 2006 [3, 9], and in Australia in which it was introduced in the examinations of the Royal Australian and New Zealand College of psychiatrists in 2004 [10]. It is used regularly in undergraduate medical education in KSA since 2014.

## Definition and Structure

R-type questions (or extended matching questions) are a type of MCQs that are rich in context; components of an R-type question are the *theme, homogenous options list* (answers), *lead-in statement, and stems* (questions inform clinical scenario or vignette), (See the provided template in Fig. 7.1 and the examples in Figs. 7.2, 7.3, and 7.4). The candidate must match the stems with the provided options; the combination of the options (answers), lead-in, and stems (question) collectively make one item that addresses one theme. It is an objective and reliable assessment tool [11].

**Theme** It is the title; examples for basic sciences are anatomical relation, innervation, blood supply, drug or pathogen class, and cell or tissue type. For clinical sciences, examples are a complaint, physical signs, laboratory tests, or drugs. The theme is useful in a way it shows to which extent the assessment is aligning with the blueprint.

**Options** The options represent the answers for the questions (the stems), each option can be selected only once, more than once, or not selected at all; it is recommended that to enlist three or more distractors (should be plausible) for each stem, the option can be composed of one word or a short sentence. In basic sciences, the list of options can be set of embryological origins, nerves, muscles, site of arterial supply, enzymes, or hormones, while, in clinical sciences, the list can be set of

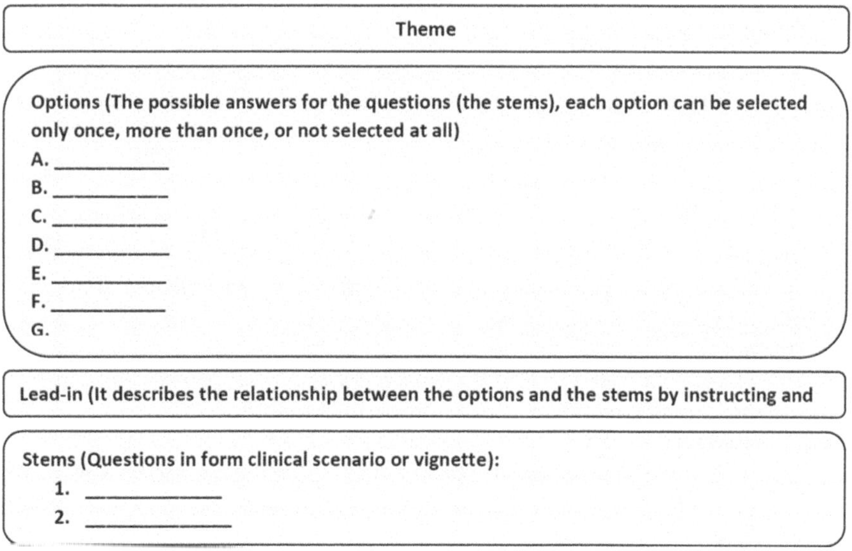


**Fig. 7.1** A template provided to guide test developers

**Theme:** Functions of the arches of the foot

**Options:**

A. Head of the talus.
B. Peroneus longus muscle.
C. Peroneus brevis muscle.
D. Plantar aponeurosis.
E. Spring ligament.
F. Tibialis anterior muscle.
G. Tibialis posterior muscle.

**Lead-in:**

Concerning the functions of supporting the arches of the foot, for each described function mentioned below, select the correct anatomical structure from the options (above) that performs that function; some of the options (anatomical structures) may not be used and some of them may be used more than once.

**Stems:**

1. Hanging the medial longitudinal arch upward.
2. Hanging the lateral longitudinal arch upward.
3. Supporting the medial longitudinal arch by binding its two ends.
4. Supporting the keystone of the medial longitudinal arch.
5. Hanging the transverse arch upward.

**Fig. 7.2** Example of a set of extended matching questions (R-type MCQs) in basic science: anatomy

**Theme:** CBC results of a patient with a sore throat

**Options:**

| | Neutrophils | Lymphocytes | Eosinophils | Basophils |
|---|---|---|---|---|
| A. | 60% | 30% | 3% | 0% |
| B. | 65% | 35% | 2% | 0.3% |
| C. | 80% | 40% | 1% | 0.2% |
| D. | 62% | 45% | 25% | 10% |
| E. | 50% | 60% | 4% | 0.1% |

**Lead-in:**

From the provided cells values of white blood cells for each patient above, select the most likely diagnosis.

**Stems:**

1. A 21-year-old male came to the emergency room with a fever and sore throat, on examination he has strawberry-like tonsils.
   **Answer: C**
2. A 16-year-old girl severely allergic to nuts, came with rash, facial swollen and redness.
   **Answer: D**

**Fig. 7.3** Example of a set of extended matching questions (R-type MCQs) in physiology

**Theme:** Cutaneous manifestations of systemic disease
**Options:**
A. Acne vulgaris.
B. Herpes zoster.
C. Infective endocarditis.
D. Lupus erythematosus.
E. Measles.
F. Vitiligo.
**Lead-in:**
From your knowledge of the skin lesions for each patient select the most likely diagnosis.

Select the correct clinical description from the mentioned below and match it to the diagnoses mentioned in the options (above). Some of the options may not be matched and some of them may be matched more than once.

**Stems:**
1. A 15-year-old boy came complaining of fever and fluid-filled lesions less than 0.5 cm in diameter on his left side of the chest along his third rib.
   **Answer: B**
2. An 18-year-old girl with pain full pus-filled lesions less than 0.5 cm in diameter all over her face since she hit puberty three years ago.
   **Answer: D**

**Fig. 7.4** Example of a set of extended matching questions (R-type MCQs) in dermatology

investigations, diagnoses, drugs, or procedures, and options are better to be short, homogenous, and clear [3, 12].

The number of options affects the psychometric quality of the item [13]. The minimum number of options can be 4 options [14], 5 options [15, 16], 6 options [1], or 7 options [17], and the maximum is up to 20 [7], 26 options [17], or 16 options [18]. Furthermore, the range in the literature is variable, from 10 to 20 [9], 5 to 26 [15, 16], 9 to 26 [19]. The number of options when increased can enhance the discrimination capacity of R-type [13]. Furthermore, the highest the number of the options the lowest probability of guessing. However, 8 options are preferred [20].

**Lead-in** In the set, there is one lead-in, which describes the relationship between the options and the stems by instructing and directing the candidate to match between them. It must be clear and shows whether the student can select the option once or more than once [7].

***Stems*** While the options are usually short, the stems are long, for they represent questions in the form of a clinical scenario or vignette. There are commonly one to two stems in each item, and there can be up to 4 stems [12]. However, the efficient use of R-type is by using fewer options (answers) and more stems (questions) [14, 21].

## Educational Impact

Students' learning is influenced by assessment, unlike A-type MCQs, which have been criticized in that they encourage superficial learning and recalling of facts [7], R-type questions encourage deep learning [9]. They can assess clinical reasoning [18, 22, 23], and the level of the competency of the candidate does not affect this capacity [24]. It is reported that when solving R-type questions, backward reasoning (i.e., confirming the diagnosis using the available investigations' results and clinical findings) is used by non-experts and forward reasoning (pattern recognition) is used by experts. Thus R-type can differentiate experts from non-experts [24, 25], and the capacity of R-type to assess clinical reasoning is higher than A-type MCQs [3]. However, assessing clinical reasoning is not necessarily depending on the selection of the assessment tool (A- or R-type MCQs) or modifying the number of options in the question, it is rather achieved by refining the stem [26]. In comparison with open-ended questions such as (short answer question), R-type question provides wider and better coverage of the content as well as domains [3].

## Psychometric Properties

R-type questions present validity evidence in the category of contents, in which the test questions represent all the learning outcomes (i.e., it is a matter of sampling). Due to the nature of the questions in which each one has a theme, the distribution of the themes (according to the learning outcomes) on a blueprint is easy [27]. It is reported that the evidence of validity when using R-type questions can be strengthened by using supportive means to the question as clinically relevant images [28]. Measuring the correlation between R-type and other types of questions is one way to present evidence of validity. It is reported that the correlation between 25 EMQs and 450 true/false questions in an exam was 0.43. In the same exam, the correlation was 0.60 with 10 short answer questions, −0.08 with 3 essays, 0.83 with 20 OSCE questions, and 0.48 with 2 long cases. The positive correlation between R-type questions and OSCE indicates the ability of R-type to assess clinical reasoning [23].

Reliability is achieved when a test yields consistent results when repeated. The scores from this test are considered reliable. R-type questions are considered reliable; a large number of questions can be introduced in a short time [17]. The internal consistency (Cronbach's alpha) is an index to measure the reliability, it ranges from 0 to 1. If the reliability of a test was below 0.5, it indicates weak reliability, above 0.5 is acceptable but the recommended score is between 0.70 and 0.90. The higher the number of questions, the higher the reliability [29], and it has been reported that about 105 questions in a test can yield reliability of 0.85, about 70 questions yield reliability of 0.79, and 52 questions can yield reliability of 0.75 [30]. Also, 100 questions of R-type questions yielded 0.80 [17]. However, increasing the questions (with a different theme for each question) seems to increase the reliability of R-type questions more than increasing the questions in each theme (or topic) [15]. The R-type questions are more reliable than A-type MCQs [9, 18, 31]. It is reported that the reliability of 240 MCQs was 0.83, while it was 0.90 for 220 questions of EMQs [32].

About discrimination index, extended matching questions are better discriminators than A-type MCQs [31, 32]. Discrimination properties show rather interesting facts: R-type questions are better in identifying good performing students, while A-type items are better in identifying poor-performing students. The possible explanation is that A-type may allow for scoring correct answers by guessing. Thus, application of "correction for guessing" by applying penalties on wrong answers in A-type has limited the guessing behavior of the students; however, it is speculated that the application of the same principle on R-Type questions may also enhance their discrimination capacity [19]. Increasing the number of options can have better effect on discrimination [8], and [13] it is reported that decreasing number of options (down from 26) can decrease the response time with little effect on the discrimination index, which allows for less time needed for each item with fewer options [21] and [20].

Regarding difficulty, the large number of options reduces the possibility of guessing [21]; however, it also increases the response time [8, 13, 14].

R-type questions are feasible and easier to be introduced, administer, and score; the student takes one and half a minute on average in each question [17]. It is also reported that 24 R-type items with 3 stems in each can be answered in 1 hour [1]. Another study found that 43 items with 11–25 options (median 14) and one stem in each can be answered in 1 hour [14], and in 1 hour, 50–54 items with 8 options and one stem can be solved [20, 21]. Furthermore, the nature of the structure of the item that is based on a theme makes it possible to generate many questions for the same theme, allowing for many versions of assessment [27]. This also can be done by changing the lead-in, which creates a new question without having to change the theme, options, or the stems [10].

**Take-Home Message**

R-type items are objective tools to assess clinical reasoning. Improving the psychometric properties depends on the number of the options as well as the stems, and increasing the number of options will enhance the discrimination index and reduce the guessing probability of the item. Yet it will increase the time required for the test. Thus, 8 options are recommended to get the ultimate use of time, discrimination, and difficulty indices. More evidence of validity can be presented by increasing the number of items up to 100 and ensuring the alignment of themes according to the blueprint.

## References


1. van Bruggen L, Manrique-van Woudenbergh M, Spierenburg E, Vos J. Preferred question types for computer-based assessment of clinical reasoning: a literature study. Perspect Med Educ. 2012; 1(4):162–71.
2. Hrynchak P, Takahashi SG, Nayer M. Key-feature questions for assessment of clinical reasoning: a literature review. Med Educ. 2014; 48(9):870–83.
3. Duthie S, Hodges P, Ramsay I, Reid W. EMQs: a new component of the MRCOG Part 2 exam. The Obstetrician & Gynaecologist 2006; 8(3):181–5.
4. Wood EJ. What are Extended Matching Sets Questions? Bioscience Education 2015; 1(1):1–8.
5. Downing SM. Threats to the validity of locally developed multiple-choice tests in medical education: construct-irrelevant variance and construct underrepresentation. Adv Health Sci Educ Theory Pract. 2002; 7(3):235–41.
6. Tweed M. Adding to the debate on the numbers of options for MCQs: the case for not being limited to MCQs with three, four or five options. BMC Med Educ. 2019; 19(1):354.
7. Wilson R, Case S. Extended matching questions: an alternative to multiple-choice or free-response questions. J Vet Med Educ. 1993; 20(3).
8. Case SM, Swanson DB. Extended-matching items: a practical alternative to free-response questions. Teaching and Learning in Medicine: An International Journal. 1993; 5(2):107–15.
9. Burton JL. How to write and how to answer EMQs. Obstetrics, Gynaecology & Reproductive Medicine. 2009; 19(12):359–61.
10. Samuels A. Extended Matching Questions and the Royal Australian and New Zealand College of Psychiatrists written examination: an overview. Australas Psychiatry. 2006; 14(1):63–6.
11. Case SM, Swanson DB. Constructing written test questions for the basic and clinical sciences. 3 ed: National Board of Medical Examiners Philadelphia; 2000.
12. Duthie S, Fiander A, Hodges P. EMQs: a new component of the MRCOG Part 1 examination. The Obstetrician & Gynaecologist. 2007; 9(3):189–94.
13. Case SM, Swanson DB, Ripkey DR. Comparison of items in five-option and extended-matching formats for assessment of diagnostic skills. Acad Med. 1994; 69(10 Suppl):S1–3.
14. Swanson DB, Holtzman KZ, Clauser BE, Sawhill AJ. Psychometric characteristics and response times for one-best-answer questions in relation to number and source of options. Acad Med. 2005; 80(10 Suppl):S93–6.
15. Dory V, Gagnon R, Charlin B. Is case-specificity content-specificity? An analysis of data from extended-matching questions. Adv Health Sci Educ Theory Pract. 2010; 15(1):55–63.
16. Al-Wardy NM. Assessment methods in undergraduate medical education. Sultan Qaboos Univ Med J. 2010; 10(2):203–9.
17. Beullens J, Van Damme B, Jaspaert H, Janssen PJ. Are extended-matching multiple-choice items appropriate for a final test in medical education? Med Teach. 2002; 24(4):390–5.
18. NAZIM SM, TALATI JJ, PINJANI S, BIYABANI SR, ATHER MH, NORCINI JJ. Assessing clinical reasoning skills using Script Concordance Test (SCT) and extended matching questions (EMQs): A pilot for urology trainees. Journal of Advances in Medical Education & Professionalism. 2019; 7(1):7.
19. Eijsvogels TM, van den Brand TL, Hopman MT. Multiple choice questions are superior to extended matching questions to identify medicine and biomedical sciences students who perform poorly. Perspect Med Educ. 2013; 2(5–6):252–63.
20. Swanson DB, Holtzman KZ, Allbee K. Measurement characteristics of content-parallel single-best-answer and extended-matching questions in relation to number and source of options. Acad Med. 2008; 83(10 Suppl):S21–4.
21. Swanson DB, Holtzman KZ, Allbee K, Clauser BE. Psychometric characteristics and response times for content-parallel extended-matching and one-best-answer items in relation to number of options. Acad Med. 2006; 81(10 Suppl):S52–5.

22. Tan K, Chin HX, Yau CWL, Lim ECH, Samarasekera D, Ponnamperuma G, et al. Evaluating a bedside tool for neuroanatomical localization with extended-matching questions. Anat Sci Educ. 2018; 11(3):262–9.
23. Wass V, McGibbon D, Van der Vleuten C. Composite undergraduate clinical examinations: how should the components be combined to maximize reliability? Medical Education. 2001; 35(4):326–30.
24. Beullens J, Struyf E, Van Damme B. Do extended matching multiple-choice questions measure clinical reasoning? Medical education. 2005; 39(4):410–7.
25. Beullens J, Struyf E, Van Damme B. Diagnostic ability in relation to clinical seminars and extended-matching questions examinations. Med Educ. 2006; 40(12):1173–9.
26. Coderre SP, Harasym P, Mandin H, Fick G. The impact of two multiple-choice question formats on the problem-solving strategies used by novices and experts. BMC Medical Education 2004; 4(1):23.
27. Bhakta B, Tennant A, Horton M, Lawton G, Andrich D. Using item response theory to explore the psychometric properties of extended matching questions examination in undergraduate medical education. BMC Med Educ. 2005; 5(1):9.
28. Vorstenbosch MA, Bouter ST, van den Hurk MM, Kooloos JG, Bolhuis SM, Laan RF. Exploring the validity of assessment in anatomy: Do images influence cognitive processes used in answering extended matching questions? Anatomical sciences education. 2014; 7(2):107–16.
29. Lukić IK, Glunčić V, Katavić V, Petanjek Z, Jalšovec D, Marušić A. Weekly quizzes in extended-matching format as a means of monitoring students' progress in gross anatomy. Annals of Anatomy – Anatomischer Anzeiger. 2001; 183(6):575–9.
30. Kreiter CD, Ferguson K, Gruppen LD. Evaluating the usefulness of computerized adaptive testing for medical in-course assessment. Acad Med. 1999; 74(10):1125–8.
31. McCoubrie P. Improving the fairness of multiple-choice questions: a literature review. Med Teach. 2004; 26(8):709–12.
32. Fenderson BA, Damjanov I, Robeson MR, Veloski JJ, Rubin E. The virtues of extended matching and uncued tests as alternatives to multiple choice questions. Human pathology. 1997; 28(5):526–32.

# Chapter 8
# Script Concordance Test

**Nurhanis Syazni Roslan and Muhamad Saiful Bahri Yusoff**

**Abstract** Script concordance test (SCT) is used to test how well learners can make decisions in unclear or uncertain situations. It lets testing real-life situations that other assessment tools do not measure well enough. The goal of this chapter is to discuss how doctors and health professionals make decisions, the construction principles related to SCT, and how to score SCT.

*By the end of this chapter, the reader is expected to be able to*

1. Understand the use of script concordance test.
2. Construct script concordance test.
3. Discuss the psychometric properties of script concordance test.

**Keywords** Clinical reasoning · Script concordance test

## An Assessment of Clinical Reasoning Process

In medical training, students are equipped to acquire theoretical knowledge, professional skills, and clinical reasoning [1]. There are many high-quality tools available to assess knowledge and skills. However, commonly used selected-response or constructed-response tools were found to have limitations in assessing clinical reasoning. Attempt to assess clinical reasoning using highly authentic case simulation such as the patient management problem (PMP) was less promising as it can only fit a limited number of cases in each assessment [2]. Growing studies have shown that ability to solve one case is a poor predictor of an individual ability to solve another problem (*case specificity*), and the higher yield in reliability is achieved by testing about two to three items per case [3].

N. S. Roslan (✉) · M. S. B. Yusoff
Department of Medical Education, School of Medical Sciences, Universiti Sains Malaysia, Kota Bharu, Kelantan, Malaysia
e-mail: nurhanis_syazni@usm.my; msaiful_bahri@usm.my


H. E. E. Gasmalla et al. (eds.), *Written Assessment in Medical Education*,
https://doi.org/10.1007/978-3-031-11752-7_8

On top of that, conventional tools failed to discriminate test takers from various clinical experiences (*intermediate dip phenomenon*) as these formats did not integrate practical experience with theoretical knowledge [4]. Available selected-response tools such as single best answer or multiple true false accept one answer. However, this may not be the case in daily clinical practice where a certain amount of ambiguity could be present that makes data interpretation neither algorithmic nor straightforward. Hence, the script concordance test (SCT) is introduced, as a standardized selected-response tool that can assess authentic ill-defined clinical scenarios [5, 6]. The SCT compares the test takers' answer with the panels of experts' answer, and it was found to have a good discriminant validity when tested in cohorts of varying clinical experience [1, 7, 8].

Theoretically, clinical reasoning is explained by the script theory from the field of cognitive psychology. When applied to medicine, script theory proposes that knowledge is structured into richly organized networks, or "scripts" that connect relevant broad and specific clinical information. "Illness scripts" are formed from the first year of undergraduate training and continuously updated, expanded, and restructured as one progresses through medical training [6]. When presented with a case, students or physicians will think using two complementary reasoning process, depending on the prior experience and complexity of the case:

(a) A nonanalytic process that very much built on pattern recognition
(b) A slower, analytical process that relies on hypothesis testing and deductive thinking [9]

## Construction Principles

1. Experts have cautioned the use of SCT as a tool to assess clinical reasoning as a whole. SCT assesses the data interpretation or hypothesis evaluation stage of clinical reasoning [9]. It is commonly used to assess data interpretation in diagnosis, investigation, treatment, and professional judgment [5].
2. Prior to constructing SCT, the test developer must carefully consider the following:

   (a) The purpose of the assessment—low-stakes or high-stakes examinations. Apart of being used as an advancement criterion, SCT has been described as one of the formative assessment tools to identify test takers who struggle with clinical reasoning process and provide feedback for curriculum review [10].
   (b) To create an assessment blueprint to identify an adequate sampling of clinical cases that impose diagnosis, investigation, or treatment challenge to the test takers. This can be achieved by doing a record keeping on challenging clinical encounter in daily practice [9].

3. Guidelines recommended that two authors who are familiar with the students and clinical contexts construct the cases. Cases are comprised of a vignette, diagnostic/investigation/treatment items, new information, and a Likert scale response (Fig. 8.1).
   (a) Vignette: The vignette should provide a short and challenging scenario for the test takers. The most important feature of the vignette is that it lends itself to various possibilities of differential diagnosis and is not definitive for one condition. This could be a simple statement of one sentence or a detailed lengthier statement. In a newer format called the evolving SCT (E-SCT), a new piece of information (expanded vignette) is also added after the first case to illustrate the evolution of the case and test candidate on the following phase of decision-making [11].
   (b) Items: As discussed earlier, these items could be task on diagnosis, investigation, treatment, or professional judgment. Hence, the items could be a set of differential diagnosis, investigation work-up, or options of treatments that one considers in solving a problem. The items should be homogenous and can range from two to five items. Similar to the recommendation made for other selected-response formats, using three items per case has been recommended to achieve a good reliability [12]. This is also compatible with the

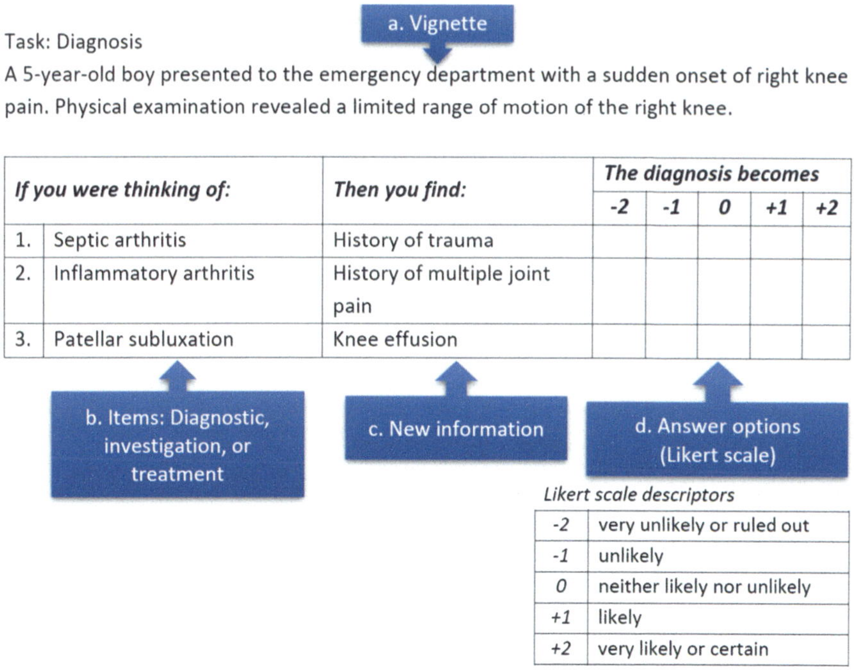


| *If you were thinking of:* | | *Then you find:* | *The diagnosis becomes* | | | | |
|---|---|---|---|---|---|---|---|
| | | | *-2* | *-1* | *0* | *+1* | *+2* |
| 1. | Septic arthritis | History of trauma | | | | | |
| 2. | Inflammatory arthritis | History of multiple joint pain | | | | | |
| 3. | Patellar subluxation | Knee effusion | | | | | |

| | |
|---|---|
| *-2* | very unlikely or ruled out |
| *-1* | unlikely |
| *0* | neither likely nor unlikely |
| *+1* | likely |
| *+2* | very likely or certain |

**Fig. 8.1** Example of a script concordance test case assessing on diagnosis

limitation of the working memory which permits a small number of working hypotheses at a time [9]. It is also important to note that each item is independently assessed and does not provide an additive information to the next item [6].

(c) New information: For each item, the authors should provide a new piece of information to assist the test takers on deciding whether the hypothesis is supported or less supported. SCT is based on the assumption that test takers with more robust illness scripts will select a similar response that is given by experts in the same scenario [9]. The new information could be a piece of history, clinical feature, or investigation result. However, to prevent cueing effect on test takers, these new information on different items should be constructed to represent various Likert responses [6].

(d) Likert scale: The Likert scale typically ranges from three to five, but five are more commonly described [13]. The descriptors varies with the task of the questions as shown in Figs. 8.1, 8.2, 8.3, and 8.4 [6]. It is important to provide suitable descriptors to each question and avoid a universal anchor, as it potentially confuses test takers and affects the response process validity [14].

4. The cases draft should be sent to at least two faculty members to review the relevance and comprehensibility of the questions [9]. The reviewers could give feedback based on the item quality grid introduced by Fournier et al. [15]. This checklist allows a reviewer to comment on the vignette (challenging, appropriate, typical, have the relevant detail, and correctly written) and the items (relevant, independent, functional new information, clear Likert scale, variable response to prevent cueing) [15]. Confusing vignette or item should be discarded or revised.

Some examples involving investigation, treatment, and judgment are illustrated as below. Note that while most of the structures are similar, the Likert scale are modified to suit the nature of the task.

Task: Investigation

Clinical vignette:
A 50-year-old female presented to the outpatient clinic with a unilateral right leg swelling for the past week. She has diabetes mellitus.

| | ***If you were thinking of:*** | ***Then you find:*** | ***The investigation becomes*** | | | | |
|---|---|---|---|---|---|---|---|
| | | | ***-2*** | ***-1*** | ***0*** | ***+1*** | ***+2*** |
| 1. | Ultrasound of the right leg | History of prolonged immobilization | | | | | |
| 2. | CT Scan of the right leg | No sign of crepitus over right leg | | | | | |
| 3. | Aspiration for culture | History of fall | | | | | |

*Likert scale descriptors*

| | |
|---|---|
| *-2* | completely unnecessary / contraindicated |
| *-1* | less useful / less indicated |
| *0* | neither less nor more useful / indicated |
| *+1* | more useful / more indicated |
| *+2* | completely useful or completely indicated |

**Fig. 8.2** An example of script concordance test case assessing problem solving on investigation

Task: Treatment

Clinical vignette:
A 60-year-old female presented to the emergency department complaining right hip pain following a fall at home. Radiograph showed neck of femur fracture. Patient is planned for an emergency right hip replacement.

| | *If you were thinking of:* | *Then you find:* | *The treatment becomes* | | | | |
|---|---|---|---|---|---|---|---|
| | | | *-2* | *-1* | *0* | *+1* | *+2* |
| 1. | Bisphosphonate | Patient has mild hypocalcemia | | | | | |
| 2. | Bipolar hemiarthroplasty | History of previous pain over the same site | | | | | |
| 3. | Starting on anticoagulant | Patient was on epidural analgesic post operatively | | | | | |

*Likert scale descriptors*

| | |
|---|---|
| *-2* | completely unnecessary / contraindicated |
| *-1* | less useful / less indicated |
| *0* | neither less nor more useful / indicated |
| *+1* | more useful / more indicated |
| *+2* | completely useful or completely indicated |

**Fig. 8.3** An example of script concordance test case assessing problem solving on treatment

Task: Research methodology

Scenario:
You would like to explore the effect of late comers to individual work productivity. You have 6 months to complete the data collection in a big private institution.

| | *If you were thinking of:* | *Then you find:* | *The method becomes* | | | | |
|---|---|---|---|---|---|---|---|
| | | | *-2* | *-1* | *0* | *+1* | *+2* |
| 1. | In depth interview | Participants have limited break time | | | | | |
| 2. | Focus group discussion | Participants freely interact with their superiors | | | | | |
| 3. | Observation | Participants are busy throughout working hours | | | | | |

*Likert scale descriptors*

| | |
|---|---|
| *-2* | completely unsuitable |
| *-1* | less suitable |
| *0* | neither suitable nor unsuitable |
| *+1* | more suitable |
| *+2* | completely suitable |

**Fig. 8.4** An example of script concordance test case assessing problem solving on professional judgment

## Panel of Experts

1. The SCT scoring relies on comparing the test takers' answer to the panel of experts' answer. A higher score indicates that the test takers are closer to the experts' script and has better data interpretation or hypothesis evaluation ability [6].
2. The questions are sent to a panel of experts for the scoring system. These panel of experts should be involved with the teaching and suit the purpose of the assessment. For example, in a certifying examination for general practitioner, the panel should represent the spectrum of subspecialties and setting across general practice [2].
3. The number of panel of experts depends on the stakes of the assessment but should be more than five to illustrate the possible variabilities of answers for each case [6]. Use of ten or more experts is associated with an acceptable reliability. As for high-stakes examination, studies have recommended using 20 experts to achieve a good reliability. Inviting more than 20 experts were found to have little gain in the psychometric properties [16].
4. Although a good number of experts should be involved, these experts do not require a training or preparation. The experts should be asked to answer all of the

items for each of the cases individually. Although they may complete the task at their convenient time, it is a good practice to answer the items under the same time constraints given to the test takers [9].

## Scoring

1. The scoring is unique as it considers the variability of responses from the panel of experts in an ill-defined case. Hence, there are several types of scoring that has been described for SCT which include the following [17, 18]:
    (a) Aggregate scoring method
    (b) Aggregate with distance method
    (c) Distance from mode method
    (d) Single answer or consensus method
    (e) Standardization method
2. The optimal scoring method for SCT remains a topic of research. However, studies found that aggregate scoring method is straightforward and provides a better score discrimination between the test takers [2, 5]. In this method, proportional credit or weightage is assigned to each of the answers given by the experts, divided by the modal value for the item [5].
3. In a hypothetical item illustrated in Table 8.1, imagine the scoring is developed by answer script of ten experts. None of the experts selected response −2 or −1; hence, test takers who selected these responses will be awarded 0 mark. Six experts selected response +1, and this has become the mode answer. For both aggregate scoring and consensus method, test takers who selected +1 will be awarded 1 mark. One expert selected response 0, test takers with this response will receive 0.16 mark (1/6) for aggregate method and 0 mark for consensus method. On the other hand, three experts selected response +2, test takers with this response will receive 0.50 mark (3/6) for aggregate method and 0 mark for consensus method.
4. A good feature of SCT item is that it should have some response variability around the modal answer, a key of its discriminatory ability (Table 8.2). An item that yields a unanimous response should be converted to a multiple-choice

**Table 8.1** Simulation of scoring using aggregate and consensus method

| Likert scale | −2 | −1 | 0 | +1 | +2 |
|---|---|---|---|---|---|
| Frequency of being selected by the experts | 0 | 0 | 1 | 6 (mode response) | 3 |
| Weightage | 0 | 0 | 1/6 | 6/6 | 3/6 |
| Points given to the test takers based on the aggregate method | 0 | 0 | 0.16 | 1.00 | 0.50 |
| Points given to the test takers based on the single answer or consensus method | 0 | 0 | 0 | 1 | 0 |

**Table 8.2** Simulation of response variability for a script concordance item

| Likert scale | −2 | −1 | 0 | +1 | +2 |
|---|---|---|---|---|---|
| Unanimous response | 0 | 0 | 0 | 15 | 0 |
| Uniform divergence response | 3 | 3 | 3 | 3 | 3 |
| Deviant response | 1 | 0 | 0 | 13 | 1 |
| Ideal variability | 0 | 0 | 1 | 12 | 2 |

question as there is only a single correct answer for it. On the other hand, an item with uniform divergence response could indicate ambiguity of the question and has a poor discriminating ability. This item should be considered to be rewritten or removed. Item with deviant response exhibits some divergence response from the cluster of responses. Guidelines recommended that this item can remain as removing it did not affect the item reliability [9].

## Assessment Utility

It is apparent that selection of assessment tools and the pursuit to achieve good psychometric properties depend on the stakes of the assessment. This concept of assessment utility encourages test developer to reflect on the importance and compromise that has to be made on validity, reliability, educational impact, cost and feasibility [19]. As for high-stakes assessment, validity and reliability are an important consideration. However, it is important to note that validity is not a property of a tool, but of the tool scores and its interpretation [20]. Using a framework discussed in Chap. 1, the test developer could look for evidence that support validity evidence or find areas for improvement (Table 8.3).

**Take-Home Messages 1. Script concordance test (SCT) is a standardized tool to assess data interpretation or hypothesis evaluation stage of clinical reasoning.**

2. SCT is an ideal tool to assess authentic, complex clinical case or professional practice where there is lack of general consensus among the experts.
3. SCT is able to compare test takers' scripts and experts' scripts and differentiate those whose script are more developed.
4. SCT can assess students up to evaluation stage in Bloom's taxonomy (C5) and Knows-How level in Miller's pyramid.
5. Studies proposed that it can be a valid and reliable tool for high-stakes assessments.
6. SCT can also serve as a formative assessment to identify areas of training, and it encourages reflection and focused discussion between novice and experts.

**Table 8.3** Description of validity evidence

| Validity evidence [20] | Potential sources in SCT |
|---|---|
| Content | Test blueprint—developed from clinical encounter<br>Training of test developer<br>Well-written case<br>In practice of item banking, good cases can be identified using item analysis. While item analysis could be less straightforward in SCT, guidelines have recommended calculation of item-total correlations. Items that produce correlation of less than 0.05 indicate a poor discriminative ability and should be considered for removal [9] |
| Response process | Familiarity of test takers with the format<br>Appropriate language<br>Use of suitable Likert scale descriptors to increase accuracy of response interpretation [14] |
| Internal structure | Sufficient number of cases and items. Studies found that 25 well-written cases of three items yields a reliability coefficient of 0.75–0.86 [2]. As for testing time, a test of 60–90 minutes was found to produce good score of reliability [9]<br>Sufficient number of experts to produce a good scoring range. Use of more than 10 experts is associated with an acceptable reliability and use of 20 experts is recommended for high-stakes assessment [16] |
| Relation to other variables | Correlational study with tools assessing similar domain. For example, a study on SCT on emergency medicine residents found that it has a good correlation with the United States Licensing Examination (USMLE) Clinical Knowledge exam [21]. |
| Consequences | Method of determining pass-fail score. The commonly used standard setting methods for dichotomous response are not suitable for SCT. Some of possible methods are Extended Angoff, subtraction of 4 standard deviation to the mean of experts rating [2], adapted Nedelsky approach [22], and standardization method [18]<br>Improvement of test takers' clinical reasoning or patient outcome |

# References


1. Subra J, Chicoulaa B, Stillmunkés A, Mesthé P, Oustric S, Bugat MER. Reliability and validity of the script concordance test for postgraduate students of general practice. Eur J Gen Pract. 2017;23(1):209–14.
2. Dory V, Gagnon R, Vanpee D, Charlin B. How to construct and implement script concordance tests: Insights from a systematic review. Med Educ. 2012;46(6):552–63.
3. Norman G, Bordage G, Page G, Keane D. How specific is case specificity? Med Educ. 2006;40(7):618–23.
4. Ramaekers S, Kremer W, Pilot A, van Beukelen P, van Keulen H. Assessment of competence in clinical reasoning and decision-making under uncertainty: The script concordance test method. Assess Eval High Educ. 2010;35(6):661–73.
5. Charlin B, Van Der Vleuten C. Standardized assessment of reasoning in contexts of uncertainty: The script concordance approach. Eval Heal Prof. 2004;27(3):304–19.
6. Charlin B, Roy L, Brailovsky C, Goulet F, Van Der Vleuten C. The Script Concordance Test: A Tool to Assess the Reflective Clinician. Teach Learn Med. 2000;12(4):189–95.

7. Ducos G, Lejus C, Sztark F, Nathan N, Fourcade O, Tack I, et al. The Script Concordance Test in anesthesiology: Validation of a new tool for assessing clinical reasoning. Anaesth Crit Care Pain Med. 2015;34(1):11–5.
8. Kania RE, Verillaud B, Tran H, Gagnon R, Kazitani D, Tran Ba Huy P, et al. Online script concordance test for clinical reasoning assessment in otorhinolaryngology: The association between performance and clinical experience. Arch Otolaryngol – Head Neck Surg. 2011;137(8):751–5.
9. Lubarsky S, Dory V, Duggan P, Gagnon R, Charlin B. Script concordance testing: From theory to practice: AMEE Guide No. 75. Med Teach. 2013;35(3):184–93.
10. Humbert AJ, Johnson MT, Miech E, Friedberg F, Grackin JA, Seidman PA. Assessment of clinical reasoning: A Script Concordance test designed for pre-clinical medical students. Med Teach. 2011;33(6):472–7.
11. Cooke S, Lemay JF, Beran T. Evolutions in clinical reasoning assessment: The Evolving Script Concordance Test. Med Teach. 2017;39(8):828–35.
12. Rodriguez MC. Three options are optimal for multiple-choice items: A meta-analysis of 80 years of research. Educ Meas Issues Pract. 2005;24(2):3–13.
13. Lubarsky S, Charlin B, Cook DA, Chalk C, van der Vleuten CPM. Script concordance testing: A review of published validity evidence. Med Educ. 2011;45(4):329–38.
14. Gawad N, Wood TJ, Cowley L, Raiche I. The cognitive process of test takers when using the script concordance test rating scale. Med Educ. 2020;54(4):337–47.
15. Fournier JP, Demeester A, Charlin B. Script concordance tests: Guidelines for construction. BMC Med Inform Decis Mak. 2008;8:1–7.
16. Gagnon R, Charlin B, Coletti M, Sauvé E, Van Der Vleuten C. Assessment in the context of uncertainty: How many members are needed on the panel of reference of a script concordance test? Med Educ. 2005;39(3):284–91.
17. Wilson AB, Pike GR, Humbert AJ. Analyzing Script Concordance Test Scoring Methods and Items by Difficulty and Type. Teach Learn Med. 2014;26(2):135–45.
18. Charlin B, Gagnon R, Lubarsky S, Lambert C, Meterissian S, Chalk C, et al. Assessment in the context of uncertainty using the script concordance test: More meaning for scores. Teach Learn Med. 2010;22(3):180–6.
19. Van Der Vleuten CPM, Schuwirth LWT. Assessing professional competence: From methods to programmes. Med Educ. 2005;39(3):309–17.
20. Cook DA, Beckman TJ. Current concepts in validity and reliability for psychometric instruments: Theory and application. Am J Med. 2006;119(2):166.e7–166.16.
21. Humbert AJ, Besinger B, Miech EJ. Assessing clinical reasoning skills in scenarios of uncertainty: Convergent validity for a script concordance test in an emergency medicine clerkship and residency. Acad Emerg Med. 2011;18(6):627–34.
22. Linn AMJ, Tonkin A, Duggan P. Standard setting of script concordance tests using an adapted Nedelsky approach. Med Teach. 2013;35(4):314–9.

# Chapter 9
# Introduction to the Psychometric Analysis

**Amal Hussein and Hosam Eldeen Elsadig Gasmalla**

**Abstract** The aim of this chapter is to describe the detailed process of exam evaluation, before and after implementing the exam. Exam evaluation starts by a qualitative review, which takes place before exam administration, and is followed by a quantitative analysis. The quantitative exam analysis is, in turn, classified into two parts: examinees' scores analysis and post-exam psychometric analysis. Qualitative and quantitative methods utilized throughout the exam evaluation process will be discussed. The chapter starts off by defining and differentiating between the three most popular theories behind the process of measurement, in this case assessment. Afterwards, the statistical methods used in exam evaluation are explained and elaborated using simple and descriptive examples.

*By the end of this chapter, the reader is expected to be able to:*

1. Describe the qualitative evaluation of exams.
2. Define and interpret the basic statistics used in analyzing examinees' scores and psychometric analysis of MCQs.
3. Interpret the basic statistics used in the quantitative analysis of exams which includes examinees' scores analysis and post-hoc exam psychometric analysis.

**Keywords** Item analysis · Item difficulty · Item discrimination index · Psychometric analysis · Reliability · Standard error of measurement

---

A. Hussein (✉)
Department of Family & Community Medicine and Behavioral Sciences, College of Medicine, University of Sharjah, Sharjah, United Arab Emirates
e-mail: amalmh@sharjah.ac.ae

H. E. E. Gasmalla
University of Warwick, Coventry, United Kingdom

Al-Neelain University, Khartoum, Sudan
e-mail: hosam.mohammed@warwick.ac.uk



H. E. E. Gasmalla et al. (eds.), *Written Assessment in Medical Education*,
https://doi.org/10.1007/978-3-031-11752-7_9

## Introduction

In medical education assessment, multiple-choice questions (MCQs) are more effectively, and thus more commonly, used in assessing the cognitive skills of undergraduate medical students [1]. Therefore, the discussion included in this chapter refers to the use of A-type MCQs rather than other question formats including modified essay questions (MEQs) and short answer questions (SAQs).

## Theories Behind Testing

The theories help to comprehend the process of measurement; those theories were developed to measure the reliability of (in our case) the assessment tool. However, there is no unified theory [2]; in this chapter, we will simplify the most renowned theories: the classical test theory, the generalizability theory, and item response theory.

### *Classical Test Theory (CTT—1968)*

It is based on understanding the notion of true, observed, and error scores: the true score ($T$) is the score that indicates the competency of the candidate in a perfect assessment, without any errors, which is an ideal situation that never happens in reality; hence, this score is not detected (by the observer). The observed score ($X$) is the actual score that is obtained by the candidate and detected or recorded by the observer. Because of possible errors, the candidate obtains the observed score when he/she is supposed to obtain the true score. Those errors are the reason that the observed score is different from the true score. This difference can be either positive, when the observed score is higher than the true score, or negative when the observed score is lower [3].

Thus, the concept of the classical test theory can be presented in the following equation: $X = T + e$; in which $E$ is the error score ($e$). Thus, reliability is expressed by the proportion of the true score to the observed score, the high proportion indicates that the true score is getting close to the observed score, which reveals minimal errors in the test. The statistics drawn from this theory include Cronbach's alpha for reliability, and item difficulty and discrimination indices. It is important to note that these indices depend on the competency/performance level of the candidates.

## *Generalizability Theory (G Theory—1972)*

It is based on the same notion of measuring the error (the difference between the true and observed scores), which is based on many factors that contribute to that error. The difference between this and CTT is that the latter considers one source of error, and it can only deal with that one source (intra-rater, inter-rater, test-retest, or internal consistency), while the G theory considers all the multiple sources of an error at once [4].

## *Item Response Theory (IRT)*

Unlike the classical test theory, the analyses driven from this theory are affected neither by the difficulty of the item nor by the ability of the group of candidates. Here, there are many statistical models. One of them is the Rasch model, a one-parameter model, which means that, in order to describe the item's characters and candidate's ability, this model uses one parameter: item difficulty [5].

**Practical Application**
**Differences between CTT and IRT**

According to CTT, if the difficulty index for an item is 0.07, it only indicates its difficulty among a certain group of candidates. If another group of candidates is subjected to the same item, the difficulty index is expected to be different. So, is this item difficult or easy? In fact, the cohort of students represents a confounding factor.

On the other hand, let us imagine introducing an easy test to a student, whose score was 85%. If we introduced another test that assesses the same contents and domains, but the test is difficult, the same student would score, say, 65%. Thus, what is the actual level of competence and performance of that student? In fact, the different levels of difficulties of the test items represent a confounding factor.

What is the actual item difficulty? What is the actual ability of the candidate? Statistics driven from CTT are sample-dependent, those driven from IRT are not. The candidates' ability and the difficulty of test items are confounding factors. On the contrary, IRT can answer this question by eliminating the confounders.

The IRT eliminates confounding factors such as the different abilities of the students by considering all the students with the same ability.

## Qualitative Evaluation of Exams

In medical education, written examinations are used as effective assessment tools that help faculty evaluate the knowledge and outcome competencies of students. Examinees' scores inform teaching faculty and curriculum developers about necessary changes that are needed to enhance the quality of instruction and/or make curricular changes. Therefore, in order to achieve the exam's intended purpose, and ensure high exam reliability and content validity, it is necessary that exam items (questions) be evaluated prior to the exam administration. Knowing that writing a good exam question is a challenge, it is not unexpected to find a few errors or flaws in some exam items. Following exam construction, a qualitative review of the individual exam items is done by a committee. This committee should include the exam writer, who is most probably the subject matter expert and course instructor, in addition to at least two other members. The role of this review committee is to evaluate the quality of the overall exam as well as its individual items. The first step of exam review would be to ensure that the exam questions align with the learning outcomes stated in the exam blueprint [6]. In other words, exam questions should assess the learning outcomes of the assessed course. Exam blueprint is an effective method of maximizing exam content validity [7, 8]. In this respect, committee members should reject to review an exam that is submitted without its blueprint.

The qualitative review of an exam is suggested to cover general as well as specific aspects of the exam. The following aspects refer to the general aspects that should be reviewed in an exam [6]:

A. Alignment of exam items with the learning outcomes stated in the test blueprint should be checked.
B. Exam items should not use negatively worded statements.
C. Medical abbreviations should be clarified the first time they are mentioned in the exam.
D. Exam items should avoid using adverbs of frequency, such as usually, sometimes, frequently, and generally.
E. Spelling, grammatical, punctuation, and capitalization errors are checked and edited.

After reviewing the general aspects in an exam, specific details are also evaluated. These details are either related to the stem of the question, or to its answer options/distractors. Below is a list of the specific issues to be reviewed by the committee:

A. Question stem is a vignette-format providing a rich context related to the examined concept.
B. Question stem includes enough information to answer the question, for example, patient's age, sex, presenting problem, medical history, followed by findings of physical examination and diagnostic tests, etc.
C. Question should be checked for clarity in relation to language.
D. Question stem, as well as distractors, should not include any cues or terms that lead to the correct answer.

E. Questions should use suitable terminology and be suitable to the level of exam takers.
F. In case the question has an attached image or figure, the reviewers should make sure that the attachment is essential to answer the question.
G. The question is answered by a single correct answer even before reading the answer options.
H. The question scenario should be followed by a clear lead-in question.
I. The lead-in question should avoid using the word "Except."
J. Answer options/distractors should be as short as possible and should not be too long.
K. Answer options should be homogeneous. For example, if the question inquires about the most appropriate treatment, then the answer options are expected to include names of drugs.
L. Answer options should avoid using the following terms: "All of the above," "None of the above," Option B&D, etc.
M. Answer options should not be overlapping; that is, one option should not be included in another option.
N. The correct answer should neither be the longest nor the shortest among all the options.
O. Question should have only one correct answer or a single best answer.
P. Distractors should be functioning, that is, plausible and close to the correct answer.
Q. All distractors should be written using the same grammatical structure.
R. All distractors should be as long as the correct answer.
S. All distractors should be scientifically correct statements.

The qualitative review of the constructed exam items is completed by the committee members who identify the problematic items. Some problems might be corrected by the committee who might themselves revise and edit some questions. Yet, other problems that are subject related are highlighted and referred to the item writer for modification and re-submission. Subsequently, the finalized version of the exam will be ready for administration among intended exam takers.

## Quantitative Analysis of Exams

Following exam administration, another review process of the exam is launched, and this pertains to a quantitative analysis of the examinees' scores and the exam psychometrics. This quantitative analysis utilizes statistical measures to inform about the quality of the exam as a whole as well as its individual items. Quantitative revision is based on the data collected from the examinees' scores on the exam.

The following section explains the quantitative exam revision process. This process includes analyzing and describing the distribution of the examinees' scores as well as specific statistical measures that are used in a post-exam psychometric analysis. Furthermore, an explanation about the calculations of these measures and their interpretations are also included.

## *Analysis of Examinees' Scores*

After exam administration, examinees' raw scores are collected and analyzed. Descriptive measures of central tendency including the mean and median scores are calculated to describe the central location of the examinees' scores. In addition, measures of variability including the standard deviation and the interquartile range are calculated to reflect the level of variation in the scores. Furthermore, a graphical presentation of the frequency distribution of the examinees' scores, using the histogram, visually illustrates the major features of the distribution of scores and informs about the appropriate summary measures that should be reported for the set of examinees' scores on an exam.

### Graphical Presentation of Examinees' Scores (Histogram)

A histogram, which is a special type of bar chart, is a graphical presentation used to display the frequency distribution of a set of scale data, in this case examinees' scores. In a histogram, scores are the values presented on the horizontal *X*-axis, while the frequency or number of occurrences of each score or a range of scores is presented on the vertical *Y*-axis. A range of scores on the horizontal axis is called a class interval (e.g., scores falling in the range 70–75). Above each class interval, is a rectangular bar, the height of which corresponds to the frequency or the number of scores that fall within that interval [9].

The shape of a histogram, showing examinees' scores on an exam, not only informs about the performance of the students on that exam, but also provides an idea about the difficulty of that exam before even discussing the findings of its psychometric analysis. Figure 9.1a is an example of a histogram showing a normal distribution of examinees' scores. The normal distribution curve is bell-shaped and indicates that the mean and median scores are equal and divide the students, based on their exam scores, into two equal groups. In other words, half of the students achieved below the mean score and the other half achieved above it. Figure 9.1b is a histogram showing a positively skewed distribution in which the majority of students achieved low scores and very few scored high on the exam. A positively skewed distribution generally indicates poor examinees' performance and possibly an exam with too many difficult items. Figure 9.1c presents a negatively skewed

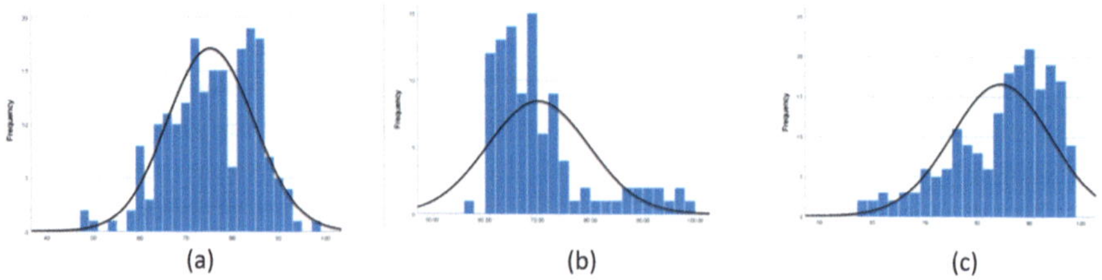


**Fig. 9.1** Histograms showing different distributions of examinees' scores. (**a**) Normal distribution; (**b**) positively skewed distributions; (**c**) negatively skewed distributions

distribution with a tail to the left side indicating that the majority of students achieved high scores and very few scored low on the exam. A negatively skewed histogram indicates an exam with relatively easy items.

## Mean and Standard Deviation (SD)

The mean score of students is the "average score," also called "arithmetic mean," which is calculated by adding up all the examinees' scores and dividing the calculated sum by the number of examinees. Standard deviation (SD) is a measure of dispersion of examinees' scores around the mean [10]. A low SD value indicates that examinees' scores form a cluster and are close to the mean, showing homogeneity in examinees' scores, while a high SD value shows a wide spread of the examinees' scores in relation to the mean, indicating variation in examinees' marks. With regard to exam evaluation, a large value of standard deviation is more preferred since it indicates that the exam was better able to discriminate between students, and thus some achieved high scores while others scored low on the exam. The mean and the standard deviation are reported as measures of location and dispersion, respectively, only when examinees' scores show a normal bell-shaped distribution. The equations for the mean and standard deviation are as follows:

$$\text{mean} = \frac{\sum xi}{n}$$

where $xi$ is each examinee's score and $n$ is the number of examinees

$$\text{SD} = \sqrt{\frac{\sum (xi - \overline{x})^2}{n - 1}}$$

where $n$ is the number of examinees; $xi$ is the examinee's score and $\overline{x}$ is the mean score.

## Median and Interquartile Range (IQR)

The median is the middle score in a set of scores, and it is also referred to as the 50% percentile. The median score divides a set of scores into two equal subsets. Therefore, the number of students achieving a score that is equal to or greater than the median score is equal to the number of students whose scores are equal to or less than the median score. When the number of students is an odd number, and their scores are arranged in ascending or descending order, then the median score will be the middle value. If the number of students is even, then two middle values in the set of ranked scores can be identified and the median will be the average of these two middle values [9].

The interquartile range (IQR) is a measure of variability that is reported with the median score. IQR is the difference between the 75th and the 25th percentile values. In other words, the IQR captures 50% of the examinees' scores and is calculated by subtracting the value of the first quartile (Q1) from the third quartile (Q3) (IQR = Q3 − Q1) [9]. A large IQR in a set of examinees' scores reflects a wide variation among the middle 50% of the scores, while a small IQR value indicates little variation.

**Example 1**
Consider the following set of scores:

| | | | | | | | | | |
|---|---|---|---|---|---|---|---|---|---|
| 64 | 94 | 76 | 81 | 88 | 72 | 80 | 92 | 71 | 63 |
| 74 | 83 | 85 | 90 | 91 | 81 | 73 | 67 | 78 | 77 |

To calculate the mean score, we add all the scores and divide by the number of scores. Therefore:

Mean = (64 + 94 + 76 + 81 + 88 + 72 + 80 + 92 + 71 + 63 + 75 + 83 + 85 + 90 + 91 + 80 + 73 + 67 + 78 + 77)/20 = 79

To calculate the median score, first we need to order the scores in ascending order. Therefore, the ordered list will be

| | | | | | | | | | |
|---|---|---|---|---|---|---|---|---|---|
| 63 | 64 | 67 | 71 | 72 | 73 | 74 | 76 | 77 | 78 |
| 80 | 81 | 81 | 83 | 85 | 88 | 90 | 91 | 92 | 94 |

After listing the 20 scores in ascending order, the rank of the median score will be $(n + 1)/2 = (20 + 1)/2 = 10.5$th ranking score. Therefore, the median score will be the average of the 10th (78) and 11th (80) ranking scores. Thus, the median value will be (78 + 80)/2 which is equal to 79.

Analysis of examinees' exam scores not only reflects the examinees' overall performance on the exam but also informs about the performance of the exam among that specific cohort of students. For example, low mean and median scores indicate a relatively difficult exam. Yet, analyzing examinees' scores is not enough to evaluate the quality of an exam. Conducting exam psychometric analysis provides a more accurate evaluation of the exam and its items.

## *Post-Exam Psychometric Analysis*

### Exam Reliability

Generally, all measurements are associated with some degree of error. In educational assessment, examinations are the tools used to measure examinees' knowledge and competence, and the error associated with examinations is called measurement error.

To simplify the definition of measurement error, let us first discuss three important related concepts in any measurement: the observed score, the true score, and the measurement error. The observed score is simply the score that is recorded by the measurement tool that is used, while the true score is the value obtained knowing

**Take-Home Message**
**Histogram interpretation**

A positively skewed distribution generally indicates poor examinees' performance and possibly an exam with too many difficult items. While a negatively skewed histogram indicates an exam with relatively easy items.

**Interpretation of mean and standard deviation**

A low mean score indicates a relatively difficult exam, while a high mean score reflects an easy exam.

A large value of standard deviation indicates that the exam was better able to discriminate between students.

**Practical Application**
**Example 1 on Excel spreadsheet**
Let us assume the following hypothetical example of students' total scores at the end of a course. The scores are presented out of 100 and we need to calculate the mean of students' scores. The following screenshot displays an excel sheet of the students' scores. To calculate the mean, we use the excel function for the average calculation of the selected scores ranging from cells C3 till C32, as shown in the spreadsheet Fig. 9.2.

Mean = AVERAGE (C3:C32)

After defining the formula and pressing the OK button, the calculated average will be displayed in the cell as 76.96.

To calculate the standard deviation of the students' scores about the mean, another excel function is selected as shown in Fig. 9.3:

Standard deviation = STDEV (C3:C32)

After defining the formula and pressing the OK button, the calculated standard deviation will be displayed in the cell as 13.84.

As shown in Fig. 9.4, to calculate the median score value, the following excel function is used:

Median = MEDIAN (C3:C32)

After defining the formula and pressing the OK button, the calculated median will be displayed in the cell as 76.36.

Now to calculate the interquartile range, we need to first calculate the score value for the first quartile (Q1), below which lies 25% of the students' scores, and then calculate the score value for the third quartile (Q3), above which lies the 25% of the students' scores. The interquartile range will then be calculated as Q3 – Q1.

As shown in Fig. 9.5, to find the value of Q1, we use the following excel function:
Q1 = QUARTILE (C3:C32; 1); where 1 indicates returning the value of Quartile 1

Similarly, to find the value of Q3, we use the following excel function (Fig. 9.5):
Q3 = QUARTILE (C3:C32; 3); where 3 indicates returning the value of Quartile 3

For the above set of data scores, Q1 = 65.96 and Q3 = 89.23

Therefore, IQR = Q3 – Q1 = 23.27

This means that 50% of the students' scores are captured in a range of approximately 23 points (between the values of 65.96 and 89.23).

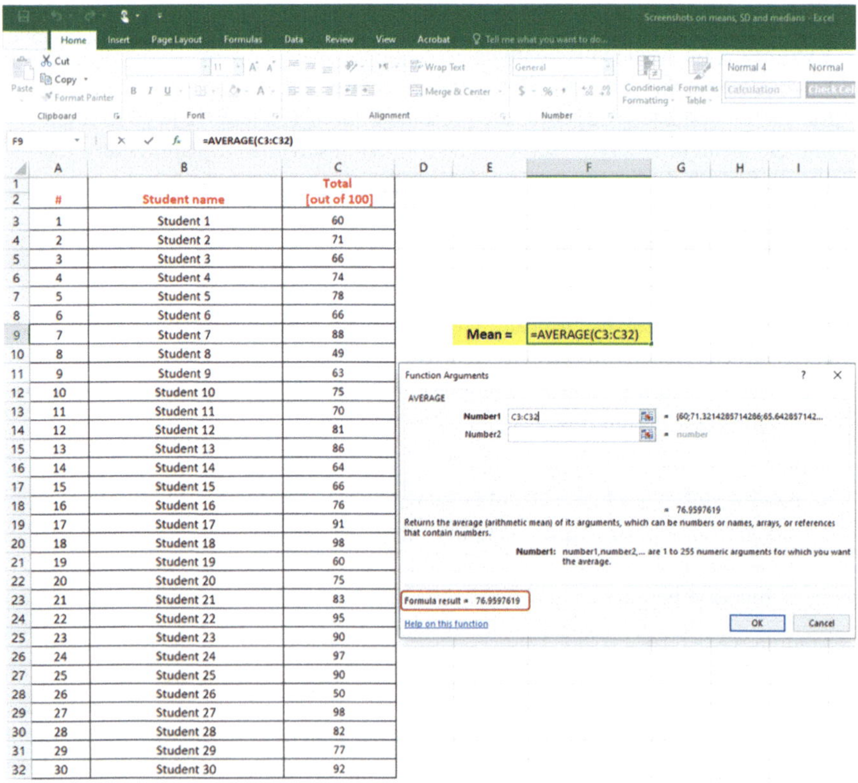


| # | Student name | Total [out of 100] |
|---|---|---|
| 1 | Student 1 | 60 |
| 2 | Student 2 | 71 |
| 3 | Student 3 | 66 |
| 4 | Student 4 | 74 |
| 5 | Student 5 | 78 |
| 6 | Student 6 | 66 |
| 7 | Student 7 | 88 |
| 8 | Student 8 | 49 |
| 9 | Student 9 | 63 |
| 10 | Student 10 | 75 |
| 11 | Student 11 | 70 |
| 12 | Student 12 | 81 |
| 13 | Student 13 | 86 |
| 14 | Student 14 | 64 |
| 15 | Student 15 | 66 |
| 16 | Student 16 | 76 |
| 17 | Student 17 | 91 |
| 18 | Student 18 | 98 |
| 19 | Student 19 | 60 |
| 20 | Student 20 | 75 |
| 21 | Student 21 | 83 |
| 22 | Student 22 | 95 |
| 23 | Student 23 | 90 |
| 24 | Student 24 | 97 |
| 25 | Student 25 | 90 |
| 26 | Student 26 | 50 |
| 27 | Student 27 | 98 |
| 28 | Student 28 | 82 |
| 29 | Student 29 | 77 |
| 30 | Student 30 | 92 |

**Fig. 9.2** Calculating the mean

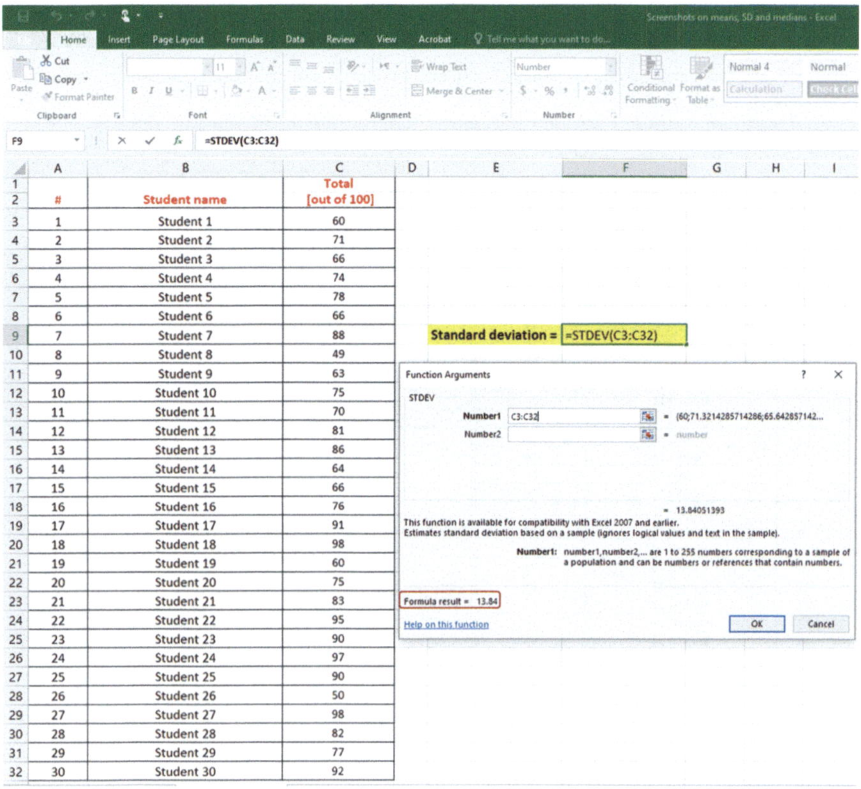


| # | Student name | Total [out of 100] |
|---|---|---|
| 1 | Student 1 | 60 |
| 2 | Student 2 | 71 |
| 3 | Student 3 | 66 |
| 4 | Student 4 | 74 |
| 5 | Student 5 | 78 |
| 6 | Student 6 | 66 |
| 7 | Student 7 | 88 |
| 8 | Student 8 | 49 |
| 9 | Student 9 | 63 |
| 10 | Student 10 | 75 |
| 11 | Student 11 | 70 |
| 12 | Student 12 | 81 |
| 13 | Student 13 | 86 |
| 14 | Student 14 | 64 |
| 15 | Student 15 | 66 |
| 16 | Student 16 | 76 |
| 17 | Student 17 | 91 |
| 18 | Student 18 | 98 |
| 19 | Student 19 | 60 |
| 20 | Student 20 | 75 |
| 21 | Student 21 | 83 |
| 22 | Student 22 | 95 |
| 23 | Student 23 | 90 |
| 24 | Student 24 | 97 |
| 25 | Student 25 | 90 |
| 26 | Student 26 | 50 |
| 27 | Student 27 | 98 |
| 28 | Student 28 | 82 |
| 29 | Student 29 | 77 |
| 30 | Student 30 | 92 |

**Fig. 9.3** Calculating the standard deviation

that a perfectly accurate measurement tool has been used. The measurement error is simply the difference between the true and observed scores. The following formula expresses the relationship between the above three concepts:

$$\text{Observed score} = \text{true score} \pm \text{measurement error}$$

In assessment, examinees' scores that are obtained after administering an exam are, in fact, the observed scores of the students. Exams are generally designed to minimize the measurement error and thus produce observed scores that are close to the true scores of students. The main problem in educational assessment is that the true scores of students are not known and therefore, quantifying the amount of error associated with the administered exams remains a necessity. Quantifying measurement errors is essential for assessing the accuracy of the examinees' results as well as for measuring exam quality.

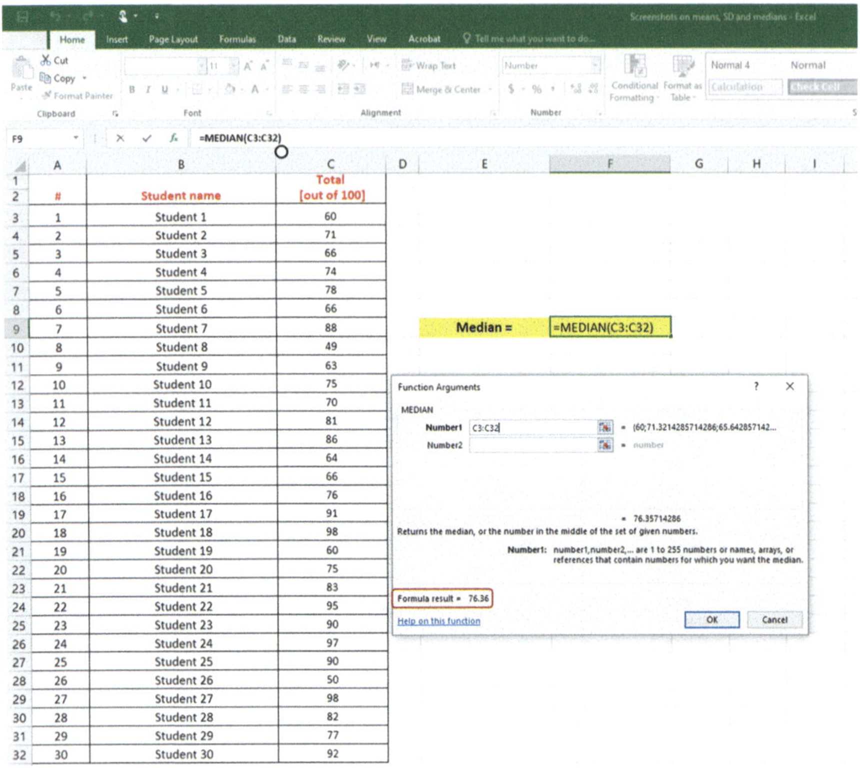


**Fig. 9.4** Calculating the median

Reliability is a measure of consistency and reproducibility of the results of a measurement tool [11]. Reliability of a measurement tool quantifies the amount of random error that is included in the measured data. The lower the measurement error in a set of data, the higher would be the reliability of the data. In other words, reliability can be defined as the proportion of the true score in the total observed score [12].

Three different methods are used to measure reliability, and these are test-retest reliability, inter-rater reliability, and internal consistency reliability.

## Test-Retest Reliability

Test-retest reliability requires the administration of the same measurement tool twice among the same group of individuals. An essential assumption here is that the time gap between the two administrations is long enough for the respondents to forget their initial answers on the first administration. Yet, the time gap should also

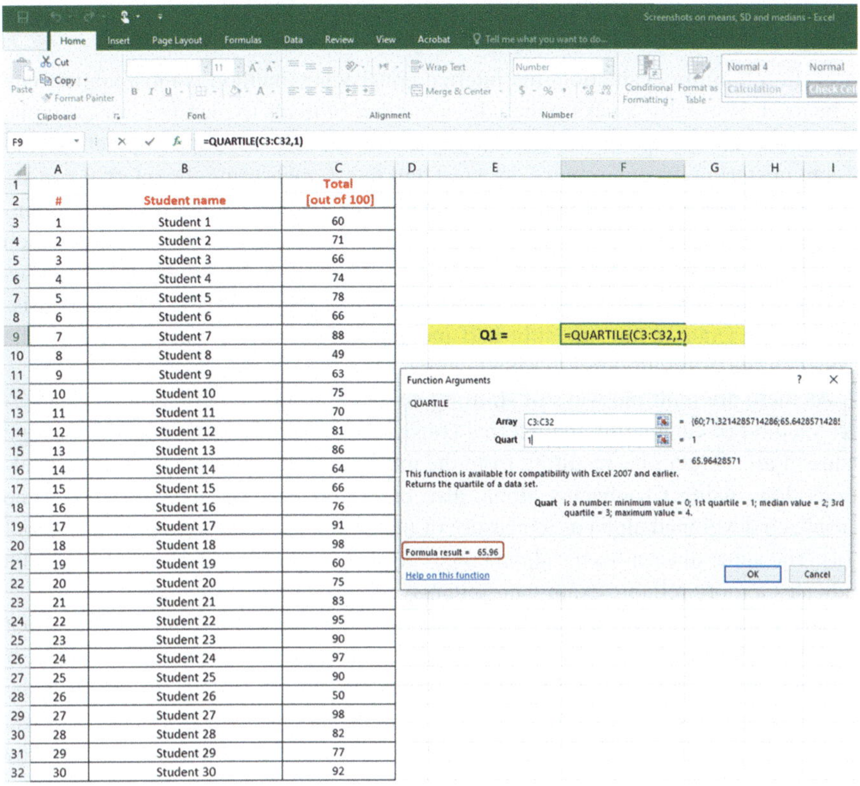


| # | Student name | Total [out of 100] |
|---|---|---|
| 1 | Student 1 | 60 |
| 2 | Student 2 | 71 |
| 3 | Student 3 | 66 |
| 4 | Student 4 | 74 |
| 5 | Student 5 | 78 |
| 6 | Student 6 | 66 |
| 7 | Student 7 | 88 |
| 8 | Student 8 | 49 |
| 9 | Student 9 | 63 |
| 10 | Student 10 | 75 |
| 11 | Student 11 | 70 |
| 12 | Student 12 | 81 |
| 13 | Student 13 | 86 |
| 14 | Student 14 | 64 |
| 15 | Student 15 | 66 |
| 16 | Student 16 | 76 |
| 17 | Student 17 | 91 |
| 18 | Student 18 | 98 |
| 19 | Student 19 | 60 |
| 20 | Student 20 | 75 |
| 21 | Student 21 | 83 |
| 22 | Student 22 | 95 |
| 23 | Student 23 | 90 |
| 24 | Student 24 | 97 |
| 25 | Student 25 | 90 |
| 26 | Student 26 | 50 |
| 27 | Student 27 | 98 |
| 28 | Student 28 | 82 |
| 29 | Student 29 | 77 |
| 30 | Student 30 | 92 |

**Fig. 9.5** Calculating the interquartile range

be short enough for the respondents not to modify their measured outcomes between the two administrations [13]. The two sets of results obtained from the two administrations are then correlated using the correlation coefficient (*r*) which ranges between −1 and +1. The value of the correlation coefficient indicates the reliability of the exam. Thus, a higher (*r*) value indicates a greater exam reliability. For example, a test-retest reliability value of +0.8 reflects a good reliable exam with an amount of 20% (1 − 0.8 = 0.2 × 100 = 20%) of random error embedded in the scores of students.

In the context of assessment, measuring test-retest reliability requires multiple administration of the same test among the same group of students. Such a requirement is impractical and imposes a serious challenge in relation to fulfilling the assumption of the test-retest reliability. Alternatively, other methods of assessing reliability are considered in the context of assessment, one of which is the internal consistency reliability.

## Internal Consistency Reliability

In exam reliability evaluation, the internal consistency method is most appropriate to be used. Normally, an exam includes a number of items to measure, for example, examinees' knowledge on a specific topic. Due to the challenge and impracticability of administering the exam twice, as a test and retest, measuring the internal consistency can be done using the split-half method. This method requires a single administration of the exam, followed by splitting the exam into two halves where each includes a random set that includes half of the exam items. Examinees' responses on the two separate halves are then correlated. Consequently, the internal consistency of an exam, using the split-half method, measures the extent to which the scores on the different items correlate with each other.

As there are multiple ways of splitting an exam into two halves, the most accurate method of calculating the internal consistency reliability is to take the average value of all correlations resulting from the multiple splits. This measure of reliability is done using Cronbach's alpha, also called coefficient alpha. In 1951, Lee Cronbach developed alpha as a measure of internal consistency of a measuring tool [14]. The value of Cronbach's alpha ranges between 0 and 1. A higher value of alpha indicates a more reliable exam whose items are correlated to each other.

The value of Cronbach's alpha informs not only about the exam reliability but also about the amount of measurement error embedded in an exam. For example, if an exam has a reliability value of 0.75, then this means that three fourth of the observed variation in the examinees' score is attributed to the examinees' abilities, or their true scores, while the rest (1 − 0.75 = 0.25 = 25%), or one fourth of the examinees' scores is due to random error.

In A-type multiple-choice exams, examinees' responses on individual exam items are recoded and changed into dichotomous responses, where a correctly answered item takes the value of 1 and an incorrectly answered item takes 0 point. In this specific situation of having dichotomous response items, Kuder Richardson-20 (KR-20) is used to measure the internal consistency reliability of an exam. KR-20 is a special type of Cronbach's alpha that is used for dichotomous response items. Similar to the Cronbach's alpha, the value of KR-20 ranges from 0 to 1 and is interpreted using the same guiding criteria (Table 9.1). The formula of KR-20 is

$$\mathrm{KR} = \frac{N}{N-1} \times \frac{V - \sum_{i=1}^{n} p_i q_i}{V}$$

where, $N$ is the number of items in the test; $V$ is the variance of examinees' raw scores; $p_i$ is the proportion of correct answers of item $i$; $q_i$ is the proportion of incorrect answers of item $i$.

**Table 9.1** Example 2—Inter-rater reliability

| | Assessors' ratings | | | |
|---|---|---|---|---|
| | Scenario A (low reliability) | Scenario B (high reliability) | | |
| Students | Dr X | Dr Y | Dr X | Dr Y |
| 1 | 87 | 79 | 91 | 90 |
| 2 | 75 | 84 | 84 | 84 |
| 3 | 82 | 86 | 70 | 71 |
| 4 | 74 | 85 | 86 | 86 |
| 5 | 92 | 81 | 65 | 66 |
| 6 | 88 | 76 | 83 | 82 |
| 7 | 68 | 77 | 78 | 78 |
| 8 | 83 | 90 | 93 | 93 |
| 9 | 85 | 85 | 85 | 84 |
| 10 | 80 | 69 | 76 | 76 |

Inter-Rater Reliability

Inter-rater reliability is also referred to as inter-observer reliability. This method of reliability assessment is used in situations when two assessors evaluate the same group of students. The scores given by the two assessors are correlated to measure their extent of agreement about the examinees' scores. Inter-rater reliability is mostly used in clinical assessments. A high value of correlation coefficient ($r$) indicates a high inter-rater reliability and thus a high level of agreement between the two raters. In the context of research conduction, this type of reliability is called equivalence reliability, and it is used to measure the reliability of a questionnaire by correlating data emerging from its translated versions [13].

**Practical Application**
**Example 2—Inter-rater reliability**

In Example 2 (Table 9.1), let us compare two scenarios, A and B, when two assessors, Dr X and Dr Y, are evaluating the same group of ten students. Let us assume that the students are being assessed on their clinical reasoning. In Scenario A, there is low inter-rater reliability about examinees' assessment as there is clear disagreement in the assessors' ratings of students. In the presence of low reliability, it would be inappropriate to use these scores. However, in Scenario B, by inspection, we can see a high level of agreement between the two assessors about the examinees' ratings which indicates a high inter-rater reliability.

## Assessing and Increasing Exam Reliability

KR-20, as a measure of exam reliability, is reported in the post-exam psychometric analysis. A higher KR-20 value indicates a better exam reliability. Different educational references have set guiding criteria for the value of Cronbach's alpha or KR-20. Here we report the criteria published by Downing [11] (Table 9.2):

Exam reliability is affected not only by the interrelationship among the items of the exam but also by the length of the exam. Therefore, it is not unexpected for a short exam to have a low KR-20 value. Therefore, to increase the value of KR-20, and improve exam reliability, the following options can be considered:

1. Adding more exam items that are related to the measured concepts results in increasing exam reliability [15].
2. Removing items that reduce exam reliability. KR-20 or Cronbach's alpha can be recalculated when each exam item is deleted, and accordingly, problematic items are identified and are excluded from the exam. Problematic items are those that, when deleted, result in higher KR-20 values.
3. Adding multiple assessment methods to the written exam creates a composite test measure that promotes the reliability of the assessment process.

**Practical Application**
**Example 3—KR-20 if item deleted (Table 9.3)**
Let us imagine an exam with a reliability measure of KR-20 = 0.794. The exam includes a total of 10 items. KR-20 is calculated when each item is deleted. Notice that KR-20 increased from 0.794 to 0.824 and 0.817 when deleting item 5 and item 6, respectively. However, KR-20 decreased when each of the other items was deleted. This indicates that items 5 and 6 are problematic items, where the deletion of which improved the exam reliability. In this case, the two problematic items should be removed from the exam and examinees' scores are recalculated.

## Item Analysis Statistics

Quantitative exam review incorporates a post-exam psychometric item analysis. Item analysis statistics provide a quality control measure of the individual exam items and of the exam as a whole. Item analysis statistics are used to improve the

**Table 9.2** General guidelines to interpret reliability coefficients of exams

| Value | Needed for…. | Example |
|---|---|---|
| ≥0.90 | Very high stakes tests | Licensure<br>Certification exams |
| 0.80–0.89 | Moderate stakes tests | End of year/course summative exam |
| 0.70–0.79 | Lower stakes tests | Formative or summative classroom assessments |

**Table 9.3** Example 3—KR-20 if item deleted

| Exam Item | KR-20 if item deleted |
|---|---|
| Item 1 | 0.752 |
| Item 2 | 0.754 |
| Item 3 | 0.766 |
| Item 4 | 0.776 |
| Item 5 | 0.824 |
| Item 6 | 0.817 |
| Item 7 | 0.762 |
| Item 8 | 0.758 |
| Item 9 | 0.772 |
| Item 10 | 0.763 |

reliability of the exam and consequently increase the validity of examinees' scores. Findings obtained from item analysis are reviewed to identify problematic exam items which are then either modified or even deleted from the exam. As a result, exam answer key is modified and finalized for final scoring of the examinees' exam responses.

Item analysis statistics include counts and proportions related to item difficulty, item discrimination index, point-biserial correlation, and distractor analysis. The following section defines each statistic and illustrates their use and interpretation using a typical example taken from a real exam.

## Item Difficulty (ID)

Item difficulty is the most basic statistic that informs about the performance of an exam question. Item difficulty is calculated for individual exam items. Item difficulty is simply the proportion (or percentage) of students who answered an exam question correctly. For example, if the ID of an exam question is 72% (or 0.72), then this means that 72% of students answered that exam question correctly. The value of the difficulty index ranges between 0% and 100%, and it directly correlates with the easiness of an exam question. Therefore, a higher ID value indicates an easier question.

According to Downing [11], in a typical exam, most exam questions should be within the item difficulty range of 0.45–0.75. The use of easy questions (ID 0.76–0.91), extremely easy questions (ID > 0.91), difficult questions (ID 0.5–0.44), and very difficult questions (ID <0.24) should be limited to essential content (Table 9.4). The use of mostly easy questions in an exam is expected to result in a negatively skewed distribution of examinees' scores. Similarly, the use of more difficult questions will result in a distribution of examinees' scores that is positively skewed. In both cases, the exam will lose its ability in identifying high- or low-performing students.

**Table 9.4** Item classification guide by difficulty and discrimination

| Item class | Item difficulty | Item discrimination (point-biserial) | Description |
|---|---|---|---|
| Level I | 0.45–0.75 | +0.20 or higher | Best item statistic; use most item in this range |
| Level II | 0.76–0.91 | +0.15 or higher | Easy; use sparingly |
| Level III | 0.25–0.44 | +0.10 or higher | Difficult; use very sparingly and only if content is essential |
| Level IV | <0.24 or >0.91 | Any value | Extremely difficult or easy; do not use unless content is essential |

Source: [11]

**Table 9.5** Calculating item discrimination

| | |
|---|---|
| Upper 27% Group | Includes high-scoring students who, based on their scores, form the top 27% of all students who sat for the exam |
| Middle Group | Includes 46% of students who achieved scores lower than those in the Upper group but above those in the Lower Group |
| Lower 27% Group | Includes low-scoring students who, based on their scores, form the bottom 27% of all students who sat for the exam |

### Item Discrimination Index

Item discrimination index (DI) is a statistical measure that determines how well an exam item was able to discriminate between knowledgeable and nonknowledgeable students, also referred to as high achievers and low achievers. To calculate the discrimination index, students are divided into three groups based on their achievement, that is their scores on the overall exam. The three groups are defined as per Table 9.5:

Discrimination index is then calculated for each item of the exam by subtracting the percentage of students in the Lower 27% Group who answered that item correctly from the percentage of students in the Upper 27% Group who answered the same item correctly. Thus, we can say that the discrimination index compares the item difficulty between the Upper 27% Group and the Lower 27% Group. For a good discriminating item, the assumption is that item difficulty is low among the Lower 27% Group, indicating a difficult item, and high among the Upper 27% Group, indicating an easy item. The following formula is used to calculate the discrimination index:

$$\begin{aligned} \text{DI} = &\ \%\text{of examinees in the Upper 27\%Group who answered item correctly} \\ &-\%\text{of examinees in the Lower 27\%Group who answered item correctly} \end{aligned}$$

The item discrimination index is a measure of item effectiveness. In other words, if an item is effective, then it is expected to be highly discriminating between students. As a result, the item is answered correctly by knowledgeable students or students who achieved high on the exam, whereas it is answered incorrectly by students with poor knowledge or low achievers. The calculated value of the discrimination index ranges between −1 and +1. Positive DI values indicate good discriminating items where examinees in the Upper Group did better on that item than the examinees in the Lower Group. On the other hand, DI values that are negative are unfavorable as they reflect better performance of the examinees who scored poorly on the exam than those who were high scorers. If the item discrimination index of an exam item is equal to zero, then this means that examinees in the Upper Group and Lower Group performed equally on that item. Items whose DI is zero or negative are considered as problematic and should be removed from the exam before final scoring is done. Generally, the minimum acceptable DI value is +0.20 [12], a higher value is even more favorable. Another classification of DI considers the value of +0.30 to indicate "good" discrimination, between 0.10 and 0.30 as "fair," and below 0.10 as "poor" [16]. A negative discrimination index indicates that the exam item is wrong and should be removed.

It is worth noting here that there is a direct relationship between item difficulty and item discrimination index. Difficult and easy exam items usually have poor discrimination power. Therefore, items with very high or very low item difficulty, generally, have low discrimination indices. Easy exam questions are usually equally answered correctly by high and low achievers. Similarly, difficult exam questions are missed by students in both groups. Therefore, when evaluating an exam item, it is essential to consider both statistics, item difficulty and item discrimination index at the same time (Table 9.2).

**Practical Application**
**Example 4—Item discrimination index**
For an exam item, let us assume that 60% of examinees in the Upper 27% Group answered the item correctly while only 20% of the examinees in the Lower 27% Group answered it correctly. This means that the item discrimination index is 60 − 20% = 40% = +0.4. Since the value of DI was positive and above 0.2, we can conclude that the item had a strong discrimination and was effective in differentiating between well-knowledgeable and poorly knowledgeable students.

### Point-Biserial Correlation

Point-biserial correlation ($r_{pb}$) is a type of correlation that is also used as an index of item discrimination. Point-biserial correlation coefficient is also calculated for each exam item. It tests the relationship between all examinees' performance on a single item and their performance on the rest of the items in the exam. In general, if an item is highly discriminating, then examinees who performed well on the exam are expected to respond correctly on that item. Similarly, examinees who performed poorly on the overall exam are expected to answer the item incorrectly.

The point-biserial correlation coefficient can range between −1 and +1, with a more favorable value that would be closer to +1. The acceptable range for a point-biserial correlation coefficient is defined as +0.30 and above, with a value of +0.40 and above indicating a good discriminator. A negative point-biserial coefficient for a question indicates an inverse relationship between that question and the whole exam. That is students who answered the question correctly did poorly on the exam. A question with a negative coefficient is either poorly written and should be removed from the exam, or has a wrong key that needs correction, or is different from the exam. Point-biserial correlation coefficient is calculated using the following formula:

$$r_{\mathrm{pb}} = \frac{\overline{Y}_1 - \overline{Y}}{S} \sqrt{\frac{n_1 - n}{(n - n_1)(n - 1)}}$$

where, $n$ = total number of examinees; $n_1$ = number of examinees who answered the question correctly; $\overline{Y}_1$ = mean score of examinees who answered the question correctly; $\overline{Y}$ = mean score of examinees who answered the question correctly; $S$ = standard deviation of examinees scores.

Distractor Analysis

Distractors are simply the incorrect options in an A-type multiple-choice question. The function of these options is mainly to distract nonknowledgeable examinees. Therefore, a distractor must be a plausible option that is reasonable to an examinee who is not highly knowledgeable, yet should be an incorrect option or at least not the best option in answering the question. The quality of a multiple-choice question depends not only on the question's correct option but also on the quality of its distractors. Item analysis statistics, which were discussed in the previous sections of this chapter, identify exam items or questions that have flaws, yet, they do not inform about the details related to that error. For example, neither the discrimination index nor the difficulty index can inform about the quality of a question's distractors. Evaluations and revisions at the item level are essential components of the post-exam psychometric analysis. Therefore, the frequency of selecting each answer option, which is called distractor analysis, is another important means of reviewing the quality of exam items.

Distractor analysis identifies distractors, or answer options, of exam items that did not function adequately, also called nonfunctional. According to Downing and

**Practical Application**
**Example 5—Item analysis statistics**
To illustrate an example related to the previously discussed concepts, let us now discuss the following condensed test report (Fig. 9.6), which displays a post-exam item analysis of an exam including a total of 51 four-option multiple-choice questions and administrated among a total of 44 examinees.

Yudkowsky [11], a nonfunctional distractor is the one that is selected by less than 5% of the examinees. Nonfunctional distractors are identified, revised, or maybe replaced before future use of the same question.

The following interpretations are made based on the results displayed in the report:

- Examinees achieved a mean score of 34.18 (SD = 7.41) and a median score of 35.50. As the mean and median scores are close, we can assume that the examinees' scores form an approximately normal distribution curve.
- The range of scores is 35, and this is the difference between the maximum score (46) and the minimum score (11) that are achieved by the examinees. Given that the total possible points is 51, and the range is 35, we can infer that the distribution of examinees' scores would show a wide spread with an expected flat histogram graph.
- The exam has good reliability with a KR-20 value of 0.85.
- The item difficulty is 81.82% for Question 1, 86.36% for Question 2, 88.64% for Question 3, 4.55% for Question 4, and 72.73% for Question 5. These results are displayed in the Correct Total % column. Accordingly, we can say that Question 4 is a very difficult question.
- Discrimination index (DI) can be calculated for the five questions by subtracting the values of the Lower 27% from the Upper 27%. Thus, for
  - Question 1: DI is 100 – 50.00% = 50% = 0.50
  - Question 2: DI is 100 – 83.33% = 16.67% = 0.17
  - Question 3: DI is 100 – 66.67% = 33.33% = 0.33
  - Question 4: DI is 8.33 – 8.33% = 0.0% = 0.00
  - Question 5: DI is 83.33 – 66.67% = 16.66% = 0.17
- We can conclude that Questions 1 & 3 have good DI (above 0.30) and Questions 2 & 5 have fair DI while Question 4 has poor DI. Question 4 is a difficult question, as indicated by a difficulty index of 4.55% and thus has a poor discriminat-

## Condensed Test Report

**Legend:** Distractors Chosen More than Correct Answer: ■

| | | | | | |
|---|---|---|---|---|---|
| **Total Possible Points:** | 51 | **Median Score:** | 35.50 | **Maximum Score:** | 46 |
| **Total Students:** | 44 | **Mean Score:** | 34.18 | **Minimum Score:** | 11 |
| **Standard Deviation:** | 7.41 | **Reliability Coefficient (KR20):** | 0.85 | **Range of Scores:** | 35 |

| No. | Question | Correct Answer | Response Frequencies A | B | C | D | E | Non Distractor | Correct Group Responses Total % | Upper 27% | Lower 27% | Point Biserial |
|---|---|---|---|---|---|---|---|---|---|---|---|---|
| 1 | Question1 | C | 4.55 | 13.64 | **81.82** | 0.00 | 0.00 | DE | 81.82 | 100.00 | 50.00 | 0.56 |
| 2 | Question2 | A | **86.36** | 2.27 | 4.55 | 6.82 | 0.00 | E | 86.36 | 100.00 | 83.33 | 0.21 |
| 3 | Question3 | C | 2.27 | 0.00 | **88.64** | 9.09 | 0.00 | BE | 88.64 | 100.00 | 66.67 | 0.61 |
| 4 | Question4 | B | 0.00 | **4.55** | 72.73 | 22.73 | 0.00 | AE | 4.55 | 8.33 | 8.33 | 0.04 |
| 5 | Question5 | D | 22.73 | 2.27 | 2.27 | **72.73** | 0.00 | E | 72.73 | 83.33 | 66.67 | 0.24 |

**Fig. 9.6** Condensed test report

ing ability among examinees. Question 4 was answered equally by the high and low performers and thus has zero discrimination index.

- Point-biserial correlation coefficients were all positive and above 0.20 except for Question 4, which had a very low coefficient ($r = 0.04$) indicating that the question is not related to the overall exam.
- Distractor analysis is displayed under the Response Frequencies Columns showing the percentage of students selecting each answer option. According to the reported values in the table, nonfunctional distractors are options A & D for Question 1, options B &C for Question 2, options A & B for Question 3, option A for Question 4, and options B & C for Question 5. These nonfunctional distractors need careful revision and modification in case we intend to use these questions in future exams. Notice that for Question 4, option C was selected by the highest proportion of students. In this case, there is a possibility that the question key is wrong. Therefore, the question should be sent back to the question writer to confirm its answer key.
- In conclusion, based on the findings of the exam's item analysis, the action plan can be set as per the following. Question 4 should be first checked for the validity of the answer key. If the answer key is correct, then the question should be deleted from this current exam and rescoring of the examinees' responses is carried out using the final validated key. Questions with nonfunctional distractors should be revised and modified to improve the questions' performance in future examinations.

**Take-Home Message**
In post-exam psychometric analysis, reliability of the exam, as measured by KR-20, is evaluated and interpreted. Item analysis statistics including item difficulty, item discrimination index, point-biserial correlation, and distractor analysis are then calculated and interpreted in order to identify problematic exam items that should be either excluded from the exam, modified and corrected, or improved for future use. Following the post-exam psychometric analysis, rescoring of the exam is done to finalize the examinees' scores.

## Standard Error of Measurement (SEM)

Standard error of measurement (SEM) is a measure of precision of the examinees' scores. In other words, SEM is an indicator of the average amount of measurement error in an exam. In simple words, SEM estimates the difference between an examinee's observed score and his/her true score. If this difference is small, this indicates that the exam is a reliable tool in quantifying the examinee's true score. However, if the value of SEM was large, then this means that the exam was not reliable in measuring the examinee's true level of knowledge. Therefore, a smaller value for SEM is highly desirable with an ideal value of zero. SEM is thus inversely proportional to the reliability of the exam. A more reliable exam is associated with lower SEM. Below is the formula used to calculate the value of the standard error of measurement:

$$r_{\text{pb}} = \frac{\bar{Y}_1 - \bar{Y}}{S}\sqrt{\frac{n_1 - n}{(n - n_1)(n - 1)}}$$

where, SD is the standard deviation of the examinees' scores; $r$ is the reliability measure of the exam calculated for a set of multiple-choice questions using the KR-20.

According to the above formula, as the value of r increases, SEM value will decrease and the opposite is also true. For a perfectly reliable exam with a reliability measure of 1, SEM will be zero. Similarly, for an exam with very poor reliability, assuming a KR-20 of zero, then SEM value will have a maximum value equal to the standard deviation of the examinees' scores. In conclusion, the standard error of measurement has a range of values between 0 and SD.

Standard error of measurement is a measure of the exam precision as it quantifies the average amount of measurement error associated with the examinees' scores. SEM is inversely related to an exam's reliability and thus affects the amount of confidence in the accuracy of the observed scores of examinees. In the presence of good quality exam items and reliable exams, SEM can be used as a method of standard setting [17]. For example, if the SEM value was 5% and the college set standard is 60%, then the value of the adjusted exam standard, or new cut-off value below which examinees are failed, would be 60 ± 5% = 55% or 65%. Students who achieved between 55% and 65% are all borderline students who might have achieved their scores due to measurement error. Therefore, scores of these students could be false positive (for those who achieved between 60% and 65%), as they passed but they deserve to fail, or false negative (for those who achieved between 55% and 60%), as they failed but deserve to pass. In order to reduce the false negative results of assessment, the college may rather decide to adopt one SEM below the set standard to generate an adjusted standard. In our example, 60 – 5% = 55% will be the new standard of the exam.

## Conclusion

In summary, examination is an essential element of assessment as well as of the teaching and learning process. Accordingly, medical schools have to make sure that the examination process is carried out with the best possible quality control measures in order to achieve valid and reliable results. Examination review and evaluation is an essential step before finalizing and reporting examinees' scores. This review represents a process that starts during exam construction and ends after exam administration. During this process, qualitative and quantitative measures are utilized.

In the first phase of the examination review process, the exam is reviewed qualitatively by a committee whose role is to check for errors embedded in individual questions and make sure that the exam as a whole is aligned with the exam blueprint addressing the course learning objectives. Following exam administration, the second phase of exam review requires quantitative statistical techniques that utilize the data generated by the examinees' raw scores. Components of the post-exam psychometric analysis include exam reliability (KR-20), difficulty index, discrimination index, point-biserial correlation coefficient, and distractor analysis. Assessment committees and faculty should carefully review all results emerging from the post-exam item analysis and discuss its implications on revising the exam items and accordingly finalizing the key for rescoring of examinees responses. Item analysis also has future implications on the assessment process. Based on the results of the item analysis, problematic items, even if removed from current exams, can be revised, modified, and improved and are ready to be used in future examinations. Therefore, item analysis is extremely effective in helping medical schools to improve their examinations and eventually build question banks that include valid and reliable multiple-choice questions ready for future use.

## References

1. Khan M, Aljarallah BM. Evaluation of Modified Essay Questions (MEQ) and Multiple Choice Questions (MCQ) as a tool for Assessing the Cognitive Skills of Undergraduate Medical Students. International journal of health sciences. 2011 Jan;5(1):39-43.
2. Schuwirth LWT, van der Vleuten, Cees P. M. General overview of the theories used in assessment: AMEE Guide No. 57. Medical teacher. 2011 Oct;33(10):783-97.
3. De Champlain, A. A primer on classical test theory and item response theory for assessments in medical education. Medical Education. 2010;44:109–117. https://doi.org/10.1111/j.1365-2923.2009.03425.x
4. Bloch R, Norman G. Generalizability theory for the perplexed: A practical introduction and guide: AMEE Guide No. 68. Medical teacher. 2012 Nov;34(11):960-92.
5. Downing SM. Item response theory: applications of modern test theory in medical education. Medical education. 2003 Aug;37(8):739-45.
6. Rudolph MJ, Daugherty KK, Ray ME, Shuford VP, Lebovitz L, DiVall MV. Best Practices Related to Examination Item Construction and Post-hoc Review. American journal of pharmaceutical education. 2019 Sep;83(7):7204-1503.
7. Ray ME, Daugherty KK, Lebovitz L, Rudolph MJ, Shuford VP, Divall MV. Best Practices on Examination Construction, Administration, and Feedback. AJPE. 2018-12;82(10):1127-32.
8. Downing SM. Validity: on the meaningful interpretation of assessment data. Medical education. 2003 Sep;37(9):830-7.
9. Daniel W, Cross C. Biostatistics: Basic Concepts and Methodology for the Health Sciences. 10th Ed ed. Singapore: John Wiley & Sons; 2014.
10. Office of Educational Assessment. University of Washington: Scorepak. Item analysis. Seattle, WA: University of Washington: Scorepak; 2005.
11. Polgar S, Thomas SA. Introduction to research in the health sciences. Seventh edition ed. Edinburgh; London; New York; Oxford; Philadelphia; St. Louis; Sydney: Elsevier; 2020.

12. Downing SM, Yudkowsky R. Assessment in Health Professions Education. New York: Taylor and Francis; 2009.
13. Nieswiadomy R. Foundations of Nursing Research. 6th ed. Pearson Health Science; 2012.
14. Cronbach LJ. Coefficient alpha and the internal structure of tests. Psychometrika. 1951 Sep;16(3):297-334.
15. Tavakol M, Dennick R. Making sense of Cronbach's alpha. Int J Med Educ. 2011-6-27;2:53-5.
16. Office of Educational Assessment. Item Analysis. University of Washington: Scorepak; 2005.
17. Hussein A, Abdelkhalek N, Hamdy H. Setting and maintaining standards in multiple choice examinations: Guide supplement 37.3 – practical application. Medical teacher. 2010 Jul 01;32(7):610-2.

# Chapter 10
# Standard Setting in Written Assessment

**Majed M. Wadi**

**Abstract** The term "standard setting" refers to the process of establishing the minimum passing score for students on a test. It is not simply a matter of arbitrarily establishing a cut score for a test; rather, it is a laborious process by which a panel determines the cut score for a specific test in a particular context.

In medication education, certifying medical students as a doctor is very critical. The decision made to graduate health-care practitioners should be based on rigorous methods to determine how much graduated doctors are safe for people's lives. For this reason, standard setting lays at the heart of the assessment. This chapter illuminates the standard setting process and discusses pertinent methods used in medical education, particularly for written tests.

*By the end of this chapter, the reader is expected to be able to*

1. Recognize concepts in standard setting and their importance in medical and health professions education.
2. Explain the common methods of standard setting in written assessment.

**Keywords** Standard setting · Angoff method · Ebel method · Borderline student

## Overview of Standard Setting

The noble goal of medical education is to graduate competent and safe physicians. As a consequence, the results of certifying safe physicians should include rigorous validity evidence on the methods used to determine graduate competencies. The standard setting process lay at the heart of these evidences [1].

Standard setting means the process of creating a cut point or boundary to ascertain examinees into either passed, failed, or borderline. To create this boundary,

---

M. M. Wadi (✉)
Medical Education Department, College of Medicine, Qassim University, Buraydah, Saudi Arabia
e-mail: m.wadi@qu.edu.sa



H. E. E. Gasmalla et al. (eds.), *Written Assessment in Medical Education*,
https://doi.org/10.1007/978-3-031-11752-7_10

many efforts should be undertaken. It is a crucial step in student assessment as a decision based on the standard has the potential effect not only on the careers of examinees but also, and more importantly, on the lives of those who would benefit from examinees certified as competent [2].

## Approaches for Assigning a Pass/Fail Status in an Evaluative Setting

There are two methods for classifying examinees as pass or fail: norm and criterion references. The following subheading highlights these techniques.

### *Criterion-Referenced Approach*

A criterion-referenced standard is an absolute standard that is calibrated against a particular level of examinee performance or against a standard, predetermined competencies on a particular examination. Each examinee is evaluated in relation to this absolute standard, regardless of the examinee group's performance on that examination [3]. In a nutshell, the methods discussed in this chapter are a form of criterion-based standard setting.

### *Norm-Referenced Approach*

The performance of an examinee is evaluated in comparison to the performance of the entire group, rather than on its own merits, which is why it is referred to as norm reference. A norm-referenced standard is one that is established relative to the performance of a group of examinees on the same examination. Thus, the standard varies according to the examinee group's performance. This may result in misinterpretation in some instances. For example, an examinee placed in a group of examinees with a low performance standard has a better chance of meeting the standard than an examinee placed in a group with a high-performance standard.

While the process of developing a norm-referenced standard is much simpler than developing a criterion-referenced standard, there is no guarantee that the standard will be equivalent between examinations, as examinee group performance may differ between examinations and cut-off scores are determined by group score distributions. Cut-off points based on norm-referenced standards are irrelevant when determining an examinee's competence or incompetence [3].

## Common Concepts in Standard Setting

**Standard Setting**
It is the methodology that is run by a panel to determine the minimum pass level (cut score) for a given test [3, 4].

**Minimum Pass Level (MPL)**
It is numerical output of the standard setting (number cut point) or boundary to ascertain examinees into either passed, failed, or borderline (minimally competent student) [5].

**Minimally Competent (Borderline) Student**
A minimally competent or borderline student is one who is just on the border of failing. This student's knowledge-base borders on the edge between competence and incompetence. The criteria for classifying students as borderline depend on several factors in a given context. These factors should be specified by the panel, for whom standard setting is assigned.

**Panel**
It is a group of medical teachers acting as judges and area experts to determine the borderline students and set the minimum pass level accordingly [4].

## General Classification of Standard Setting Methods

- *Test-centered standards* are those derived from hypothetical decisions based on the test content. In these methods, a group of expert judges set the standard by reviewing the items in the test and deciding on the level of examinee performance on these items that will be considered just adequate for demonstrating competence. Methods included in this category are as follows:
  - The Angoff method [6]
  - The Nedelsky method [7]
  - The Ebel method [8].
- *Examinee-centered standards* are those derived from reviewing the performance of examinees or a similar group prior to making judgments about what constitutes borderline performance between competence and incompetence. Methods included in this category are as follows:
  - The borderline group method [9]
  - The contrasting group method [9]

## Common Methods of Standard Setting in Written Assessment

### *The Angoff (1971) Method*

The Angoff method is commonly regarded as the most popular method of standardization. It is appropriate for both written and performance assessment. This method is based on defining and determining the features of a "borderline" examinee, that is, a marginally competent person on the edge of passing or failing. This activity should be done by a group of experts or seniors who are familiar with the specific population of students for whom the standard setting has been established. There are many variants of this method. However, for the purpose of this book and to make this method simple and understandable, we will discuss the classical Angoff method.

**Steps of Angoff Method**

1. *Defining the borderline students*

A panel of judges will first gather to discuss the qualities of a "borderline" examinee, that is, someone who is marginally competent but on the edge of passing or failing. They should be told to think of an example from the intended students' population.

2. *Review and rate test items*

The first item is read aloud by one of the judges to begin the item review. The reader, followed by the other panel members, estimates how well a borderline applicant will perform on that item. Each judge is asked to consider a sample of minimally competent persons, say 100, and estimate the proportion of these individuals who would properly answer the item. Note that the difference between "will perform" and "should perform" needs to be stressed and considered by the panel. Each new item is judged in a clockwise rotation.

3. *Record the rate*

For each item, it is possible to record the rating either by hand or with the use of an excel sheet or even Google's online form.

4. *Review the rating and coming to consensus*

If considerable gaps (more than 20%) exist between the judges' judgments after they have all given their separate judgments on all of the test's questions, a group discussion may be performed to attempt to explain why such large variances exist. Judges now have the option to amend their earlier decisions independently if they so desire.

5. *Calculate the cut-off score point*

Using the Excel sheet is the appropriate and easy way to calculate the cut-off point. It is done by calculating the average of means of all test item across all raters

**Table 10.1** Record of test items rating by the panel

| Questions | Judge 1 | Judge 2 | Judge 3 | Judge 4 | Judge 5 | Mean |
|---|---|---|---|---|---|---|
| Item 1 | 50 | 60 | 55 | 65 | 60 | 48.5 |
| Item 2 | 75 | 80 | 70 | 85 | 77 | 64.8 |
| Item 3 | 90 | 85 | 85 | 95 | 80 | 73.0 |
| Item 4 | 55 | 50 | 55 | 60 | 45 | 44.8 |
| Item 5 | 70 | 80 | 77 | 70 | 65 | 61.2 |
| Average of means | 58.5[a] | | | | | |

[a]This the cut-off point (minimum pass level)

(judges). Table 10.1 is an example. This average represents the cut-off point for making pass/fail decisions.

## *Nedelsky (1954) Method*

This method was developed for multiple-choice questions, in which a panel evaluates each MCQ item and its distractors and assigns a score to each option based on how frequently minimally competent (borderline) students choose each option. The average rating for each MCQ item is calculated, and then the average rating for all items is added.

**Steps of Nedelsky Method**

1. Create a rating form (you can use an online form) that includes the serial number of the MCQ and its associated option, as well as a method for marking the key answer (using star for example).
2. Create a new file that contains the MCQ items (either word or PPT file).
3. Assemble a panel (5–10 senior medical educators who are subject-matter experts).
4. Brief the panel on the specific task assigned to them.
5. Define the minimally competent (borderline) student's criteria.
6. Display each MCQ item and request that the panel open the form.
7. Begin the session by asking the panel to rate each option as 1 if it is difficult to get the borderline student's attention and 0 if it is easy to get his/her attention.
8. The critical response should be designated as 1.
9. Add the sum of the distractors assigned as 1 to each MCQ item.
10. Estimate the MPL for each item using the following formula: MPL is equal to $1/m$ ($m$ is the number of the distractors that were assigned as difficult).

**Practical Application**

If we have a test with 30 MCQs, the Minimum pass index of each item should be added.

Example: Minimum pass index of item 1 + Minimum pass index of item 2 + … + weight of item 30

Suppose that we got the value of 22.98 for all 30 items.

The cut-off point (the minimum pass level MPL) for the Nedlesky method is then calculated by dividing MPI by the number of MCQs.

The MPL = 22.98/30 × 100 = 76.6%

11. Finally, a grand average for all items is calculated by adding the MPL of each item and dividing it by the total number of items (Table 10.2).

## *The Ebel (1972) Method*

Two characteristics of each item should be considered in the Ebel method (Ebel 1972): difficulty (easy, medium, difficult) and relevance (essential to know, important to know, acceptable, or nice to know). The judges then estimate the proportion of borderline examinees who will be able to respond to these types of questions (after their classification in two dimensions matrix).

**Steps of Ebel Method**

Two tasks in the Ebel method should be completed sequentially. The first task is to classify test items according to two dimensions: difficulty and relevance; the second

**Table 10.2** Example of Nedelsky method

| Items | Options | Judge 1 | Judge 2 | Judge 3 | Judge 4 | Judge 5 | Average |
|---|---|---|---|---|---|---|---|
| Item 1 | Option a | 0 | 1 | 1 | 1 | 0 | 0.38 |
| | Option b[a] | 1 | 1 | 1 | 1 | 1 | |
| | Option c | 1 | 0 | 1 | 0 | 1 | |
| | Option d | 0 | 0 | 1 | 1 | 1 | |
| | *1/difficult options* | 1/2 | 1/2 | 1/4 | 1/3 | 1/3 | |
| | *Minimum pass index* | 0.5 | 0.5 | 0.25 | 0.33 | 0.33 | |
| Item 2 | Option a | 1 | 1 | 1 | 0 | 1 | 0.36 |
| | Option b | 1 | 0 | 0 | 1 | 1 | |
| | Option c[a] | 1 | 1 | 1 | 1 | 1 | |
| | Option d | 0 | 1 | 0 | 1 | 0 | |
| | *1/difficult options* | 1/3 | 1/3 | 1/2 | 1/3 | 1/3 | |
| | *Minimum pass index* | 0.33 | 0.33 | 0.50 | 0.33 | 0.33 | |

[a]Key answer

task is to rate each item by estimating the percentage of borderline examinees who will answer each item correctly.

**First task: classification of test items into two dimensions; difficulty and relevance**

This task could be done by the same panel who will rate each item in the second task, or it could be done by another independent panel

1. Create a two-dimension matrix classifying each item in terms of difficulty (easy, medium, difficult) and relevance (essential, important, acceptable, questionable) (Table 10.3).
2. Regarding difficulty, it could be determined based on the previous data of item—if item already taken from a question bank or used again. The criteria of difficulty based on item analysis are as follows:

   - Easy (0.80–0.99)
   - Medium (0.45–0.79)
   - Hard (0.0–0.44)

   If data are not available to categorize item, difficulty could be estimated by the consensus of the panel.
3. Regarding relevance, classification should be done by the assigned panel for this task. Consensus should be reached to classify each item. If consensus discussion is infeasible, roughly if 50% raters agreed on an item with a two-dimension, it should be considered by this classification.
4. Present the end product of this task as three-column Table 10.4 as the following:

**Second task: rating of test items by the panel**

1. Now either the same panel or another independent panel should rate each test item by estimating (minimum pass level, MPL) how many of borderline students will answer this question. The rating form will like the following (Table 10.5):
2. Calculate the average of MPL rating for each item (Table 10.6).

**Table 10.3** Example of the two-dimension classification of the test items in the Ebel method

| Items | Relevance difficulty | Easy | Medium | Hard |
|---|---|---|---|---|
| Item 1 | Essential | | | |
| | Important | | | |
| | Acceptable | | | |
| Item 2 | Essential | | | |
| | Important | | | |
| | Acceptable | | | |
| Item 3 | Essential | | | |
| | Important | | | |
| | Acceptable | | | |

**Table 10.4** The end product of item classification in the Ebel method

| Items | Difficulty category | Relevance category |
|---|---|---|
| Item 1 | Easy | Essential |
| Item 2 | Medium | Important |
| Item 3 | Easy | Acceptable |
| Item 4 | Hard | Important |
| Item 5 | Hard | Important |

**Table 10.5** Rating of test item by the panel in the Ebel method

| | Classification | | Judge 1 | Judge 2 | Judge 3 | Judge 4 | Judge 4 |
|---|---|---|---|---|---|---|---|
| Items | Difficulty category | Relevance category | 45% | 50% | 60% | 45% | 55% |
| Item 1 | Easy | Essential | 50% | 70% | 70% | 50% | 45% |
| Item 2 | Medium | Important | 70% | 35% | 45% | 70% | 60% |
| Item 3 | Easy | Acceptable | 35% | 45% | 55% | 35% | 70% |
| Item 4 | Hard | Important | 45% | 50% | 58% | 45% | 58% |
| Item 5 | Hard | Important | 45% | 50% | 60% | 45% | 55% |

3. After getting MPL, provide re-distribution of items based on a two-dimension Table 10.7.
4. If you get more than one item in a cell, calculate the average of MPL for items in that cell (Table 10.8).
5. Covert the percentage into weight and calculate the weighted mean for each raw (Table 10.9).
6. Calculate the raw passing score by summing of weighted means.
   $0.57 + 1.58 + 0.69 = 2.85$
7. Get the passing score (cut-off point) of the whole test by the percentage of the sum of item weighted means over the number of items.
   $\text{MPL} = 100\% \times 2.85/5 = 57\%$

**Take-Home Message**

- While developing standards requires considerable effort, it is well worth it when used to certify safe medical doctors.
- Although there are several standard setting methods available, the Angoff method is the most popular and straightforward to use.
- Training judges is the most critical step in any standard setting process.
- There is no a gold standard setting method. For each test and its context, a standard setting method could be appropriate.
- All steps in performing standard setting should be appropriately documented as evidence to support the validity of decision making of test results.

**Table 10.6** Calculating the average of MPL

| | Classification | | Judge 1 | Judge 2 | Judge 3 | Judge 4 | Judge 4 | Average |
|---|---|---|---|---|---|---|---|---|
| Items | Difficulty category | Relevance category | 45% | 50% | 60% | 45% | 55% | 51.00% |
| Item 1 | Easy | Essential | 50% | 70% | 70% | 50% | 45% | 57.00% |
| Item 2 | Medium | Important | 70% | 35% | 45% | 70% | 60% | 56.00% |
| Item 3 | Easy | Acceptable | 65% | 80% | 70% | 60% | 70% | 69.00% |
| Item 4 | Hard | Important | 45% | 50% | 58% | 45% | 58% | 51.20% |
| Item 5 | Hard | Important | 45% | 50% | 60% | 45% | 55% | 51.00% |

**Table 10.7** Re-distribution of items after getting classification and MPL

| | Relevance | | |
|---|---|---|---|
| Difficulty | Easy | Medium | Hard |
| Essential | Item 1 (57%) | | |
| Important | | Item 2 (56%) | Item 4 (51.2%)<br>Item 5 (51%) |
| Acceptable | Item 3 (69%) | | |

**Table 10.9** Calculate the weighted means for each raw

| | Relevance | | | |
|---|---|---|---|---|
| Difficulty | Easy | Medium | Hard | Weighted mean |
| Essential | Item 1 (57%) | | | $1 \times 0.57 = 0.57$ |
| Important | | Item 2 (56%) | Item 4 + Item 5 (51.1%) | $1 \times 0.56 + (2 \times 0.51) = 1.58$ |
| Acceptable | Item 3 (69%) | | | $1 \times 0.69 = 0.69$ |

**Table 10.8** Making the average of MPL if there are more than one item in a cell

| | Relevance | | |
|---|---|---|---|
| Difficulty | Easy | Medium | Hard |
| Essential | Item 1 (57%) | | |
| Important | | Item 2 (56%) | Item 4 + Item 5 (51.1%) |
| Acceptable | Item 3 (69%) | | |

## References


1. Gasmalla HEE, Tahir ME. The validity argument: Addressing the misconceptions. Medical Teacher. 2021;43(12):1453-5.
2. Wiliam D. Meanings and Consequences in Standard Setting. Assessment in Education: Principles, Policy & Practice. 1996;3(3):287-308.
3. Bandaranayake RC. Setting and maintaining standards in multiple choice examinations: AMEE Guide No. 37. Medical Teacher. 2008;30(9-10):836-45.
4. Yudkowsky R, Downing SM, Tekian A. Standard setting. Assessment in health professions education. Vanderbilt Avenu, New York: Routledge; 2019. p. 86-105.

5. De Champlain AF. Standard Setting Methods in Medical Education. In: Swanwick T, Forrest K, O'Brien BC, editors. Understanding Medical Education. West Sussex, UK: Wiley Blackwell; 2018. p. 347-59.
6. Angoff WH. Scales, norms, and equivalent scores. In: Thorndike RL, editor. Educational measurement. Washington DC: American Council on Education; 1971. p. 508-600.
7. Nedelsky L. Absolute grading standards for objective tests. Educational and Psychological Measurement. 1954;14(1):3-19.
8. Ebel R. Essentials of educational measurement Englewood Cliffs, NJ: Prentice-Hall; 1972.
9. Livingston SA, Zieky MJ. Passing scores: A manual for setting standards of performance on educational and occupational tests. Princeton, NJ: Educational Testing Service; 1982.

## *Further Reading*

Bandaranayake, R. C. (2008). Setting and maintaining standards in multiple choice examinations: AMEE Guide No. 37. Medical Teacher, 30(9–10), 836–845. https://doi.org/10.1080/01421590802402247

Ben-David, M. F. (2000). AMEE Guide No. 18: Standard setting in student assessment. Medical Teacher, 22(2), 120–130. https://doi.org/10.1080/01421590078526

De Champlain, A. F. (2018). Standard Setting Methods in Medical Education. In: Swanwick, T., Forrest, K. and O'Brien, B. C. (eds.), Understanding Medical Education. West Sussex, UK: Wiley Blackwell, pp 347–359.

Yudkowsky, R., Downing, S. M. & Tekian, A. (2019). Standard setting. In, Assessment in health professions education. Vanderbilt Avenu, New York: Routledge, pp 86–105.

# Chapter 11
# Progress Testing in Written Assessment

**Mona Hmoud AlSheikh, Ahmad Alamro, and Majed M. Wadi**

**Abstract** Progress testing (PT) is a special written test used to assess the progress of all students enrolled in an academic program toward achieving the cognitive component of the program learning outcomes. All students at all academic levels sit for this exam concurrently at regular intervals. It is used in medical and health professions education (HPE) as a tool to track the knowledge growth of HPE students during their learning process of a program. The purpose is to assist students in understanding what is expected of them at the end of the program and in identifying their knowledge gaps.

*By the end of this chapter, the reader is expected to be able to*

1. Comprehend the concept of PT and the rationale behind it.
2. Recognize the process of designing, implementing, and evaluating PT.

**Keywords** Progress testing · Cognitive development · Curriculum monitoring · Knowledge gaps, Assessment for Learning

M. H. AlSheikh (✉)
College of Medicine, Imam Abdulrahman Bin Faisal University, Dammam, Saudi Arabia
e-mail: msheikh@iau.edu.sa

A. Alamro
Qassim University, Buraydah, Saudi Arabia
e-mail: ah.alamro@qu.edu.sa

M. M. Wadi
Medical Education Department, College of Medicine, Qassim University, Buraydah, Saudi Arabia
e-mail: m.wadi@qu.edu.sa



H. E. E. Gasmalla et al. (eds.), *Written Assessment in Medical Education*,
https://doi.org/10.1007/978-3-031-11752-7_11

## Overview of Progress Testing

Progress testing (PT) is a longitudinal assessment scheme that is designed to give feedback to the learner, the educator and the curriculum manager. PT entails administering a standardized written test toward the cognitive learning outcomes at the level of the end of the program and implemented at regular intervals [1]. In health professions education (HPE), PT is used as an assessment tool that measures the knowledge growth of HPE students over their training during undergraduate and postgraduate years. The students at all levels take this exam simultaneously. Because the PT is linked to graduation cognitive competencies, the results and feedback help students understand what is expected of them and identify their knowledge gaps. For academic staff, PT is used to monitor student learning and curriculum development [2] and is being considered a possible academic management and monitoring tool [3]. It is also a curriculum-independent assessment tool used to track HPE students' cognitive development—both fundamental and applied knowledge—throughout their program [4].

## The Concept of PT

PT is a comprehensive written examination that is rigorously designed to assess the knowledge and cognitive competencies of HPE student [5, 6]. The test comprises multiple-choice items ranging from 150 to 300 A-type MCQs per test. Each MCQ is a scenario-based question with four options and "I don't know" as the fifth option. The presence of an "I don't know" option allows students to professionally acknowledge their knowledge gaps and urge students not to guess [7]. All students take the assessment at the same time, at least once a year and up to four times a year [5]. Recently, several programs started to use another written format in the PT as well as clinical assessment modalities such as OSCE [8]. Discussing the other formats of PT is beyond the scope of this chapter (Fig. 11.1).

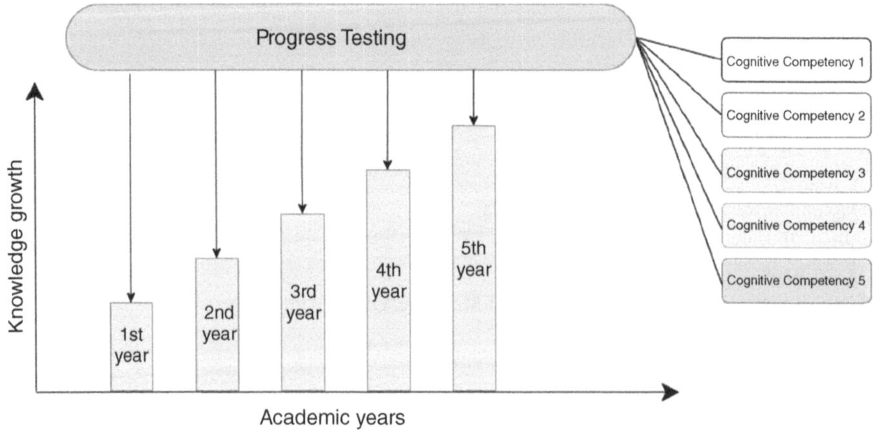


**Fig. 11.1** The concept of PT

## The Rationale for PT

When problem-based learning (PBL) was introduced as a teaching strategy in medicine, educators expressed concern about the need for an appropriate assessment of student learning that is aligned with PBL learning outcomes. This resulted in the invention of PT by Maastricht University in 1977 to ensure that the desired knowledge learning outcomes of undergraduate education were met and could be quantified clearly [1].

There are several advantages of PT. For instance, it acts as an ongoing assessment of HPE students' cognitive development, promotes long-term memory, monitors and evaluates the program, and benchmarks the program with other HPE schools/colleges [9]. Additionally, it can be used to prepare students for the HPE licensure examination [10], and the results of PT could generate longitudinal data that predict the future performance of HPE students after graduation [11]. Another primary goal of PT is to alleviate assessment-induced stress. The perceived stress caused by traditional high-stakes final exams was found to be significantly reduced when students undergo PT regularly [12, 13]. Studies found that PT inhibits the rote memorization as a strategy for exam preparation and helps students develop strategies for deep learning [13–15].

The application of PT varies among different countries around the globe. Box 11.1 shows summarized these variations.

**Box 11.1 Variations of Applying PT**

- The origin of exam construction and its blueprint is developed locally at school level or centrally at national or regional level [4, 16].
- Number of PT items (60, 150, 200, and 300 items per test) [17].
- Number of options per item (two, three, four, and five) [1].
- The approach of scoring procedure (the penalty for guessing by minus score or zero) [7].
- The used standard setting procedure (Angoff or other procedures) [18].
- The frequency of administrating PT per academic year (quarterly, biannually, and annually) [6].
- Whether the PT is compulsory or optional [6].
- Whether PT is summative or formative [19].
- The analysis theory (classic test theory vs. item response theory) [20].

## Development of PT

Apart from whether PT is locally or centrally governed, the authors will shed light, in the following subsection, on the practical steps to develop PT that would be suitable for any level.

## *Formulating a Central Committee for PT*

The presence of an independent central PT committee is crucial to ensure that the PT is developed rigorously, is a curriculum independent tool, and its items reflect the intended knowledge and cognitive competencies [5, 6]. The members of this committee should include a wide range of content experts in all basic and clinical disciplines. It should include HPE educationists to review the test items based on the appropriate guidelines of test item construction and make sure that items were crafted carefully. The crucial role of HPE educationists is to design a comprehensive PT blueprint which has many dimensions as will be explained in the subsequent paragraphs.

The main roles of the PT central committee are the following:

1. Determining the features of the PT in terms of its items number, frequency of administration, whether the test is obligatory or optional for students, and whether it is formative or summative
2. Designing a holistic and comprehensive PT blueprint
3. Suggesting the suitable guideline for test items construction
4. Recruiting good test item writers
5. Training test item writers
6. Suggesting the appropriate standard setting for the test
7. Determining the scoring criteria for the test results
8. Selecting the suitable media to announce PT results and give feedback to students
9. Suggesting the suitable form of the PT report be sent to participating schools
10. Determining the item-banking software and procedure

## *Designing PT Blueprint*

The PT blueprint should be designed expansively to include all aspects of test items starting from the item origin of scientific discipline, passing through its purpose, and finally its link to the desired intended cognitive learning outcomes.

Upon determining the number of items in PT, these items are tabulated in quota form to match the intended blueprint [16]. The following are the criteria that should be clearly specified in developing the PT blueprint:

1. The exact number and percentage of items per body system/disciplines-based/process and clinical presentations
2. The area of competencies (diagnosis, investigation, management, prognosis, and communication)
3. The matching of each PT item to the used framework of the intended learning outcomes

### *Test Item Format*

The PT could be done using any written assessment tool, and, in some countries, they used clinical formats such as OSCE. The most suitable written format is A-type MCQ—scenario-based MCQ—with a lead-in question and four plausible options including the right answer and "I don't know" as the fifth option [6]. The inclusion of an "I don't know" option enables students to properly admit their knowledge gaps, while also encouraging students to avoid guessing.

The value of the PT depends on the test items' quality, so using an item with high quality is important to ensure the validity and reliability of the interpretation. The scenario (vignette) should be crafted meticulously to test the application of knowledge and higher cognitive domains. Rubrics have been designed to judge the suitability of items to be included in a PT [21].

PT requires a huge pool of multiple-choice items. A national item bank can be created for that purpose. Alternatively, schools can subscribe to an international bank and follow a blueprint based on national qualifications for medicine to create the PT exam. National and international partnerships can reduce the burden of item construction and item banking for individual institutions [22].

### *Scoring of PT*

There are two methods for PT scoring. One strategy is to assign points for correct responses and zero points for incorrect responses, as well as the "I don't know" response. The other approach is identical to the previous one, except that it penalizes students who guess and select the incorrect option because the "I don't know" option includes a window for admitting ignorance of knowledge [7].

## PT Feedback for Students and Participating Schools

The analysis of PT could be directed to several aspects. The scores of PT can be analyzed to measure the following:

- Cognitive growth of each student in each scientific discipline and expected competencies from a medical/health-care graduate (e.g., diagnosis, treatment, and others).
- The cognitive growth is quantified as an average at different levels: comparison of students with his/her cohort of students at the school level, national level (the average of all students in the same level at participating schools in PT). It is expected that the highest growth in basic knowledge occurs between the first and second year in comparison to students at clinical levels, while the growth in the clinical knowledge is vice versa [23].

- Benchmark student cohort performance with other medical colleges or with the national average as a Key Performance Indicator of the quality of teaching and learning [24].
- Benchmark performance on each subject with other medical colleges or the national average as a curriculum monitoring tool (Fig. 5).
- Analyze the performance of the student cohort on each item for the purpose of item quality evaluation (Fig. 4).
- Each student receives a personalized detailed feedback on the learning outcomes achieved, those attempted, and those missed (Fig. 6).

## Take-Home Message

PT is a standardized written test to determine the cognitive growth of all students at regular intervals during their learning process.

PT promotes long-term memory and deep learning strategies and alleviates exam-related stress.

PT supports monitoring and evaluation of the program and benchmarks the program with other programs.

PT could be used to prepare students for the HPE licensure examination, and the results of PT could generate longitudinal data that predict the future performance of HPE students after graduation.

Developing PT requires establishing a central PT committee to design a comprehensive blueprint and set the guideline for item construction, standard setting, and scoring.

PT could be done locally at HPE school level or in collaboration with other schools at national or even regional and international levels.

## References

1. Vleuten CPMVD, Verwijnen GM, Wijnen WHFW. Fifteen years of experience with progress testing in a problem-based learning curriculum. Medical Teacher. 1996;18(2):103-9.
2. Matsuyama Y, Muijtjens AMM, Kikukawa M, Stalmeijer R, Murakami R, Ishikawa S, et al. A first report of East Asian students' perception of progress testing: a focus group study. BMC Medical Education. 2016;16(1):245.
3. Findyartini A, Werdhani RA, Iryani D, Rini EA, Kusumawati R, Poncorini E, et al. Collaborative progress test (cPT) in three medical schools in Indonesia: The validity, reliability and its use as a curriculum evaluation tool. Medical Teacher. 2015;37(4):366-73.
4. Muijtjens AM, Schuwirth LW, Cohen-Schotanus J, van der Vleuten CP. Differences in knowledge development exposed by multi-curricular progress test data. Advances in Health Sciences Education. 2008;13(5):593-605.
5. Wrigley W, Van Der Vleuten CP, Freeman A, Muijtjens A. A systemic framework for the progress test: strengths, constraints and issues: AMEE Guide No. 71. Medical teacher. 2012;34(9):683-97.

6. Dion V, St-Onge C, Bartman I, Touchie C, Pugh D. Written-Based Progress Testing: A Scoping Review. Academic Medicine. 2021.
7. McHarg J, Bradley P, Chamberlain S, Ricketts C, Searle J, McLachlan JC. Assessment of progress tests. Medical Education. 2005;39(2):221-7.
8. Pugh D, Bhanji F, Cole G, Dupre J, Hatala R, Humphrey-Murto S, et al. Do OSCE progress test scores predict performance in a national high-stakes examination? Medical Education. 2016;50(3):351-8.
9. Schauber S, Nouns ZM. Using the cumulative deviation method for cross-institutional benchmarking in the Berlin progress test. Medical Teacher. 2010;32(6):471-5.
10. Norman G, Neville A, Blake JM, Mueller B. Assessment steers learning down the right road: Impact of progress testing on licensing examination performance. Medical Teacher. 2010;32(6):496-9.
11. Schuwirth LW, van der Vleuten CP. The use of progress testing. Perspectives on medical education. 2012;1(1):24-30.
12. Pugh D, Regehr G. Taking the sting out of assessment: is there a role for progress testing? Medical Education. 2016;50(7):721-9.
13. Chen Y, Henning M, Yielder J, Jones R, Wearn A, Weller J. Progress testing in the medical curriculum: students approaches to learning and perceived stress. BMC Medical Education. 2015;15.
14. Albanese M, Case SM. Progress testing: critical analysis and suggested practices. Advances in Health Sciences Education. 2016;21(1):221-34.
15. Yielder J, Wearn A, Chen Y, Henning MA, Weller J, Lillis S, et al. A qualitative exploration of student perceptions of the impact of progress tests on learning and emotional wellbeing. BMC Medical Education. 2017;17(1):148.
16. Ricketts C, Freeman A, Pagliuca G, Coombes L, Archer J. Difficult decisions for progress testing: How much and how often? Medical Teacher. 2010;32(6):513-5.
17. Reberti AG, Monfredini NH, Ferreira Filho OF, Andrade DFd, Pinheiro CEA, Silva JC. Progress Test in Medical School: a Systematic Review of the Literature. Revista Brasileira de Educação Médica. 2020;44.
18. Bandaranayake RC. Setting and maintaining standards in multiple choice examinations: AMEE Guide No. 37. Medical Teacher. 2008;30(9-10):836-45.
19. Kerfoot BP, Shaffer K, McMahon GT, Baker H, Kirdar J, Kanter S, et al. Online "Spaced Education Progress-Testing" of Students to Confront Two Upcoming Challenges to Medical Schools. Academic Medicine. 2011;86(3):300-6.
20. Bhakta B, Tennant A, Horton M, Lawton G, Andrich D. Using item response theory to explore the psychometric properties of extended matching questions examination in undergraduate medical education. BMC Medical Education. 2005;5(1):9.
21. Janssen-Brandt XMC, Muijtjens AMM, Sluijsmans DMA. Toward a better judgment of item relevance in progress testing. BMC Medical Education. 2017;17(1):151.
22. Finucane P, Flannery D, Keane D, Norman G. Cross-institutional progress testing: feasibility and value to a new medical school. Medical Education. 2010;44(2):184-6.
23. Görlich D, Friederichs H. Using longitudinal progress test data to determine the effect size of learning in undergraduate medical education – a retrospective, single-center, mixed model analysis of progress testing results. Medical Education Online. 2021;26(1):1972505.
24. Muijtjens AM, Timmermans I, Donkers J, Peperkamp R, Medema H, Cohen-Schotanus J, et al. Flexible electronic feedback using the virtues of progress testing. Medical Teacher. 2010;32(6):491-5.

## *Further Reading*

Vleuten, C. P. M. V. D., Verwijnen, G. M. & Wijnen, W. H. F. W. (1996). Fifteen years of experience with progress testing in a problem-based learning curriculum. Medical Teacher, 18(2), 103–109. https://doi.org/10.3109/01421599609034142.

Wrigley, W., Van Der Vleuten, C. P., Freeman, A. & Muijtjens, A. (2012). A systemic framework for the progress test: strengths, constraints and issues: AMEE Guide No. 71. Medical teacher, 34(9), 683–697.

# Chapter 12
# How Written Assessment Fits into the Canvas of Programmatic Assessment

**Muhammad Zafar Iqbal and Mona Hmoud AlSheikh**

**Abstract** By the end of this chapter, the reader is expected to be able to

1. Describe the fundamental principles of programmatic assessment.
2. Describe the conceptual and theoretical frameworks that underpin programmatic assessment.
3. Identify the practical suitability of programmatic assessment in the medical curriculum.
4. Design programmatic assessment using the provided practical tips.

**Keywords** Written assessment · Programmatic assessment · Assessment for learning

## Traditional Assessment and Its Contemporary Challenges

Medical education continuously strives to improve assessment standards so that our training programs produce safe and competent physicians. To optimize the evaluation of student competence, several standardized and nonstandardized assessment tools have been tried and tested in the past and the efforts continue. However, the conventionally used assessment tools are rather subjective, situation specific, and have a variable impact on learning within and across different educational contexts [1]. Moreover, almost all assessment tools have their own limitations due to their compromised quality indicators such as validity, reliability, acceptability, and

M. Z. Iqbal (✉)
School of Physical and Occupational Therapy, Faculty of Medicine and Health Sciences, McGill University, Montreal, QC, Canada

M. H. AlSheikh
College of Medicine, Imam Abdulrahman Bin Faisal University, Dammam, Saudi Arabia



H. E. E. Gasmalla et al. (eds.), *Written Assessment in Medical Education*,
https://doi.org/10.1007/978-3-031-11752-7_12

educational impact [2, 3]. In other words, no assessment tool alone is perfect; every tool has a contextually restricted applicability and variable impact on learning [4].

To better conceptualize the limitations of assessment tools, let us take multiple-choice question (MCQ) as a working example and see how single shot assessment fails to comprehensively assess learners. As we know, MCQ is an objective type of assessment that comprises of a well-constructed scenario (stem) and a question (lead-in), followed by four or five multiple options that include one correct/best answer and distractors. Well-constructed, thoughtful, and clinical scenario-based MCQs can be used to measure higher-order cognition, problem-solving, and critical thinking skills [5, 6]. Although MCQs have multiple reported utilities, this objective assessment tool has some limitations. Most MCQ exams tend to focus only on assessing memorization and regurgitation of knowledge instead of assessing learners' higher-order cognitive, problem-solving, and critical thinking skills. This limitation has primarily been attributed to the poorly constructed questions as the assessors may not be trained enough to design proper MCQs. Moreover, MCQs cannot be used to assess psychomotor skills of the learners, which has remained a longstanding limitation of MCQs. Even if MCQs were to be perfectly designed and implemented, this assessment tool still has an inherent pitfall of fragmenting theoretical knowledge into small chunks. Although it is the assumption that combining performance of learners in MCQs with other clinical exams (i.e., OSCE) can provide a full picture of clinical competence, this is not true as confirmed by Kane's validity framework studies [7]. Furthermore, a good performance in the MCQ-based exam does not necessarily mean that the learners will be able to transfer the theoretical knowledge to clinical contexts [8]. Finally, almost all assessment tools, including MCQs, can cover only one level of Miller's pyramid; there is no tool that can magically assess learners at all levels of Miller's pyramid in one go [7, 9, 10]. More or less, similar kinds of issues can be noticed in other assessment tools (e.g., OSCEs, extended matching questions, structured oral examinations).

Now we want to draw the attention of the readers toward the pitfalls of the traditional assessment approach commonly practiced in medical schools, that is, end-of-semester/course assessment. The aim of these assessments is to measure the performance of the learners against minimum predefined standards. If a learner fails to meet these standards, then he/she is expected to retake the entire exam until he/she meets the required standards. Some medical schools also have an additional comprehensive assessment (final exam) at the end of each academic year, which is essential to pass in order to qualify for the next academic year or to graduate from a professional program. Although this classical assessment approach has served us well in the past, a scope for improvement is there because of several limitations. A major concern with the traditional assessment system is that students mostly rely upon learning and revisions prior to the block/semester exams. This just-in-time learning promotes short-term memorization and superficial learning, resulting in poor retention and translation of knowledge to clinical practice [11]. The forgetting curves from psychology suggest that learners tend to forget 50% of the learned content only after a few weeks of assessment [12]. Moreover, the traditional assessment might promote poor learning behaviors among learners as passing the course/semester becomes their main incentive to learn [13]. Another serious deficit of the traditional assessment system is that only pass/fail decision (with or without grades) is usually handed over to the learners at the end of a semester or academic year with no guidance or detailed information that can help them improve or bridge their knowledge and skill gaps. Unfortunately, our education and training practices are deprived of feedback, which is a documented, powerful source of learning [14]. These thought-provoking arguments have led the education community to rethink how we should conceptualize assessment in medical education. Probably it is time to look for an alternative approach that is not merely an assessment *of* learning but also serves as an assessment *for* learning. One such approach is the programmatic assessment that we aim to discuss in greater detail below.

## What Is Programmatic Assessment?

Programmatic assessment is a novel concept and a systematic effort toward an integrated evaluation of medical learners. Programmatic assessment is carefully selecting and deliberately arranging different forms of assessment throughout the training program to optimize learning and assessment [9]. With time, the chosen assessment methods within the programmatic assessment are continuously evaluated and modified for educational purpose. Unlike the traditional approach where a single assessment is used to make pass/fail decisions, multiple purposeful assessments (both standardized and nonstandardized) are used, each of which serves as a data point within a programmatic assessment program (Fig. 12.1). In this novel approach, the

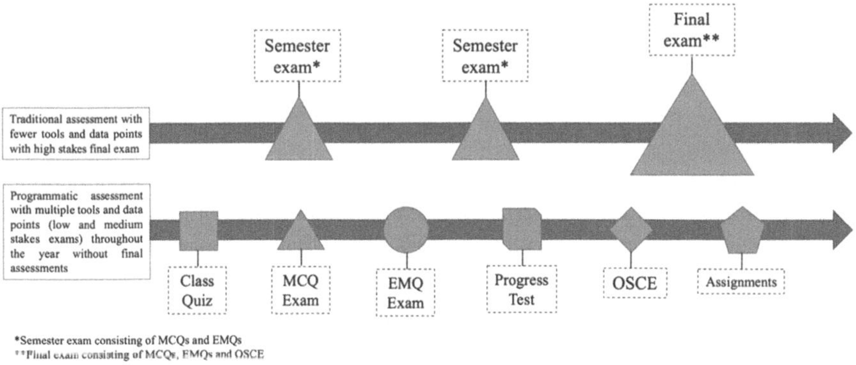


**Fig. 12.1** Traditional versus programmatic assessment

important pass/fail decisions are based on the comprehensive information that is recorded across different data points throughout an academic year. The basic idea is to replace the high-stakes, stressful semester and final exams in undergraduate training with multiple low-stakes assessments [15].

## Why Programmatic Assessment?

As discussed earlier, most traditional assessment methods in medical education are good for measuring certain domains, aspects, or competencies but are blind to others. The traditional assessment gives a snapshot of learners' competence at a particular stage in their training that remains a part of archives for the rest of the training period [7]. The programmatic assessment offers an opportunity to comprehensively assess learners' higher-order cognition, soft and psychomotor skills [16]. The information collected at multiple data points using diverse assessment methods maximizes the credibility, validity, and reliability of the inferences made, which makes programmatic assessment a "fit for purpose" approach [9]. In other words, programmatic assessment helps superimpose results from different tools to achieve a high resolution, big picture of learners' overall competence level. It is similar to subjecting a patient to various types of imaging techniques (X-ray, MRI, ultrasound, angiogram) to visualize the pathology from different angles, hoping that each imaging modality will cancel the pitfalls or blind spots of others in order to make a more reliable conclusion about the diagnosis. In research language, the idea of the programmatic assessment process can be compared to quantitative research where larger sample size is taken to minimize the error, or to qualitative research where data from different sources is triangulated to reduce bias, improve methodological rigor, and increase the depth of study findings. In crux, multiple assessments combined within programmatic assessment complement each other and provide holistic information that is richer and more valuable than the sum of individual assessments. This holistic assessment *of* learning has been found useful in overcoming the limitations of individual assessment tools that are commonly used in traditional assessment.

Another convincing feature of programmatic assessment that remains missing in traditional assessment is its potential to support learning (assessment for learning). The provision of constructive feedback is the cornerstone of the programmatic assessment approach [17]. In principle, each assessment must be twinned with formative, comprehensive, and narrative feedback that can help learners regulate their learning and improve performance. This means that the feedback should afford the learners to analyze and identify gaps in their learning, seek support when necessary, and develop a concrete action plan to fill these gaps [18]. Thus, programmatic assessment is also "assessment *for* learning" [11]. Some of the characteristic features of programmatic assessment are given below.

## Characteristic Features of Programmatic Assessment

1. Programmatic assessment is a systematic combination of multiple assessment tools that are grouped by carefully considering their strengths and weakness.
2. Programmatic assessment follows a continuous and longitudinal path during which learners' progress is recorded at each data point.
3. In programmatic assessment, the decision on learners' competence is based on the information collected and triangulated from different low-stakes assessments.
4. The reliability of the decisions on learners' competence is directly proportional to the depth, rigor, and comprehensiveness of the information collected during multiple low-stakes assessments.
5. In programmatic assessment, portfolios must be used to record information so that a rich and holistic assessment of competence can be ensured.
6. The information collected at each data point (assessment) should be meaningfully embedded within the feedback to drive learning.
7. Special attention should be paid to identify learners who are less motivated to receive and productively use feedback.
8. Ensure that the feedback loop is closed all the time. It means that the feedback should not be unidirectional. Teachers should also seek feedback from learners on how they can improve learners' learning experiences.
9. Programmatic assessment advocates scaffolding autonomy and accountability among the learners by gradually replacing structured and controlled assessments with self-regulated assessment and reflection practices.
10. The high-stakes final evaluation (pass/fail) decision should be made by an expert committee by carefully taking into account the rich information collected from multiple data points.

## Theoretical Underpinning of Programmatic Assessment

The theories that underpin the principles of programmatic assessment are *constructivist theory*, *social constructivist theory*, and *cognitive development theory* [19]. Below we briefly explain the relevance of these theories in the context of programmatic assessment.

The theory of constructivism suggests that learning is not a linear but an active, complex, and nonlinear process. In the constructivist approach, a learner makes meanings of the experiences on his/her own by internalizing and retaining new knowledge and linking it to prior information [20]. A learner constructs the information or knowledge by *processing* information instead of *consuming* it. In simple words, the constructivist theory suggests that knowledge is similar to a building construction where new floors are built onto the existing floors that provide them anchorage. This scaffolding of knowledge is, however, complex and is also influenced by social interactions between individuals. According to social constructivist theory, social processes have a critical role to play in the deep learning and cognitive development of individuals [21]. The social interactions between individuals (learners and assessors in the case of programmatic assessment) provide a venue for the individuals for shared meaning-making that is fundamental to effective learning. These social interactions not only help individuals to build new knowledge but also help the learners reconstruct their conceptual understandings. Thus, the social and collaborative setting afforded by the programmatic assessment creates various meaningful opportunities for the learners to learn new knowledge, build upon previous knowledge, and revisit their conceptual understandings [19].

Another important theoretical underpinning is the concept of dynamic assessment. Unlike traditional static assessment, dynamic assessment within programmatic assessment focuses on learners' future development through assistance (feedback). Vygotsky [22] and Feuerstein et al. [23] are of the view that it is more valuable to recognize how learners respond to feedback than merely recording what they can do at a certain time point. Therefore, the emphasis should not only be on assessing what learners have learned in the past but to think what and how they can learn in the future. This concept is in line with cognitive development theory, which is an important theoretical tenet of programmatic assessment [19]. A key concept of cognitive development theory is the zone of proximal development, which can be defined as the distance or gap between the actual and desired competence of the learners [24, 25]. The zone of proximal development is a cognitive conflict zone that occurs when learners' existing conceptualizations about the world clash with new information. It has been advocated that the conflicting thoughts serve as a starting point for the learners to reframe their understanding of the world as well as of themselves as learners [24]. Programmatic assessment demands assessors to make use of learners' zone of proximal development while providing constructive feedback so that the gap between their actual and desired level of competence can be bridged.

**Practical Application**

*Exercise:* You are the Chair of the assessment committee in your medical school. The Dean of your medical school has called a meeting of the assessment committee to share his concerns over the insufficiency of the traditional assessment. He explains to the committee that despite conducting multiple training workshops for the faculty, the exam quality is not improving. MCQs and EMQs are still testing lower-order cognition and OSCE stations are testing knowledge instead of clinical skills. He wants you to design a proposal on how to develop and implement programmatic assessment in your school's training program so that the assessment practices can be optimized. We want you to think and try to answer the following questions: How will you approach this task? What resources would be needed to design a plan? What institutional facilitators and barriers do you foresee in the implementation process?

Constructive feedback positioned around the zone of proximal development may also afford learners to self-regulate their learning by setting their own learning goals and learning strategies, and by evaluating their own performance [26].

## Practical Tips to Design and Implement Programmatic Assessment

This is probably the most difficult question to answer, and it explains the reason why the implementation of programmatic assessment has lagged in several contexts. Below we provide some practical tips that may help the readers aiming to implement programmatic assessment in their institutes in a systematic way.

### *Determine the Desired Competencies*

Determine the competencies that learners will be expected to achieve and against which the learners will be assessed during training. In programmatic assessment, selecting a competency framework is important to make a collective sense of multiple low-stakes exams and measure the progress of the learner in a specific competency. The selected framework will then provide a lens for the assessment committee to make a high-stakes decision by interpreting the data recorded across various assessment points. For instance, if *effective communication* is one of the desired competencies, then information from multiple assessment sources (e.g., OSCE, mini-CEX, multisource feedback) will be used in aggregate to make a high-stakes decision on whether the learner has successfully achieved the desired level of competence in communication skills or not.

For the selection of a competency framework, it is important to consider the affordances and limitations of the national regulatory bodies as some agencies make it mandatory for the medical schools to follow and implement a standardized competency framework. A novel approach is designing assessment around the professional tasks that are expected to be performed by the learners proficiently and independently after graduation. These professional tasks are known as entrustable professional activities (EPAs). EPAs have already been successfully used in multiple health professional domains to design and implement teaching and assessment strategies. As the description of EPAs is beyond the scope of this chapter, we recommend the readers to consult AMEE Guides 99 and 140 [27, 28] to further understand the philosophy of EPAs.

## Design an Assessment Plan

Design a master assessment plan consisting of a battery of tests or assessment tools that will be used to assess the level of learners' competence. In this master plan, the assessment tools should be mapped against each competency with clear instructions on which data point will contribute toward assessment of which competency. The selection of the assessment tools for each competency should be judicial, purposeful, and valid. For instance, to assess *clinical reasoning* of the learner, there should be a clear justification of why selected tools are more appropriate than other assessment tools. It does not matter if the chosen tool is standardized or nonstandardized as long as it is suitable for assessment of what you are aiming to assess. For instance, if the purpose of assessment is to target the "knows how" level on Miller's pyramid, then written objective assessment (MCQs, EMQs, SEQs) would be a better fit. However, if the purpose of assessment is to target "does" level, then prefer nonstandardized tools (mini-CEX, DOPs, MSF) over standardized tools (MCQs, EMQs, OSCEs). In most cases, a reluctance has been observed in preferring nonstandardized assessment tools because of the potential bias, which is understandable [29]. To avoid such bias, multiple subjective judgments should be used in combination to make a holistic judgement.

**Remember**
Involve teachers and students from the very beginning and develop a shared understanding of what programmatic is, why it is useful, and how it will be implemented.Involve learners actively and give them ownership to promote life-long learning and learner agency.

## Determine Time Points and Frequencies of Assessment

Determine at which stages in the curriculum (program) the low-stake assessments will take place and what will be the frequency of assessments to assess a particular competency. The higher will be the stakes, the more robust will be the information required to make the decisions. In certain cases, some competencies (e.g., communication skills, leadership skills, teamwork) develop over a period of time and it might not be possible to assess them in one particular course or academic year. In such cases, a longitudinal assessment might serve the purpose, meaning that the data points will then be spread across multiple courses or academic years [30]. For instance, to assess clinical reasoning, five MCQs (3rd year), two OSCE stations (one in 4th year, one in 5th year), two mini-CEX (one in 4th year, one in 5th year), and one multisource feedback (5th year) can be used as longitudinal data points. The final high-stakes decision on learners' clinical reasoning competence will be made by collectively making sense of the information received from these data points at the end of the 5th year of training.

## *Develop a Culture of Constructive Feedback*

"Nothing stimulates learning more than high-quality feedback" (p296) [31]. Since feedback is the essence of programmatic assessment, sufficient feedback opportunities should be provided to the learners on their performance so that they can steer their learning to optimally achieve the desired competence level. Note that the usefulness of the feedback depends upon its quality and richness, the credibility of the feedback provider, and follow-up practices to observe if the feedback was useful for the learner. These attributes can only be achieved if teachers and learners have a meaningful relationship and both parties truly value the importance of feedback.

## *Promote Mentorship Program*

It has been observed that feedback is often used meaningfully when given in an informal, socially comfortable way [32]. One good example of such a platform is mentor-mentee meeting. A mentor is a respected teacher who has a trust-based relationship with the learner. Sharing the assessment and feedback information with mentors and seeking their support in developing and executing the learning plan has been advocated as an effective strategy. In this approach, the control lies in the hands of the learners as they plan the meetings, self-evaluate their learning, and design future learning plan by using the assessment and feedback information. Here mentors' role is to probe, ask questions, stimulate deeper reflection, and support learners both personally (to some extent) and professionally (to the maximum extent). Mentoring program, however, is resource-intensive and enough faculty members might not be available to uptake the role of mentors. In such cases, pairing learners with senior peers might be a useful alternative option.

## *Evaluate and Adjust the Master Plan*

Similar to a curriculum, programmatic assessment evolves over time; it needs timely evaluation and continuous adjustment [31]. It is possible that the actual assessment plan may not function as expected. For instance, you may encounter poor exam reliability, teacher or learner dissatisfaction, insufficient recourses, or power. It is also possible that there are gaps or redundancies in assessment. For instance, either multiple tools are assessing the same knowledge, or some knowledge and skills are not assessed at all. In such problematic circumstances, it will be vital to systematically re-evaluate and iteratively revise the master plan by seeking support from all relevant stakeholders (administration, teachers, learners, department chairs, committees). It is also highly recommended to put a data gathering system in place that receives information from multiple sources such as pre- and post-exam analysis, student feedback reports, teacher reports, student performance in licensure exams, and survey reports. These information sources will then help the stakeholders to pinpoint the exact issues that need to be addressed in the revised master plan.

**Remember**
Normalize frequent feedback culture.Mind your context. Keep the assessment plan flexible and fit for purpose.Invest in both formal and informal faculty development programs.

## *Plan and Conduct Faculty Development*

Shifting to programmatic assessment is a gruesome process as it demands a cultural and attitudinal change in thinking about assessment, which is not a piece of cake. It is highly possible that the faculty might not consider themselves ready for this drastic change or they might have misconceptions about the novel assessment approach [33]. Another potential issue could be the inability of the faculty to provide constructive feedback. In such cases, faculty development has shown promising results in helping teachers internalize and understand the value of programmatic assessment and in developing their skillset to provide effective feedback [34]. Therefore, a dedicated training program for the faculty could immensely help in streamlining the implementation of programmatic assessment.

**Practical Application**
*Exercise:* Your institute is following programmatic assessment and written quiz test is being used as one of the tools to assess the learners' progress. To improve the formative exam quality, students are asked to take a short survey after each exam. Last semester's survey results were presented to the assessment committee in which students frequently complained that quiz tests are not helping them in their learning as their teachers are not giving them useful feedbacks. In fact, these quiz tests have become an additional source of stress because most students presume them as summative assessments. The Dean of your medical school is concerned and as the head of medical education department, she has asked you to devise a plan on how to train the faculty on conducting good quality quiz tests and giving constructive feedback. How would you approach this task? What strategies will you use to help the teachers learn these important skills?

## Take-Home Messages

1. Programmatic assessment is a novel and systematic way to optimize assessment *of* and *for* learning. There is a plethora of research that suggests that programmatic assessment works well in overcoming some of the challenges faced in traditional assessment.
2. The transition from traditional to programmatic assessment, however, is a time-taking process as it requires a major change in attitudes, policies and practices. Effective, responsive, and supportive leadership is the key to successful implementation of programmatic assessment (top-down approach).
3. Faculty development has a crucial role to play in successful implementation of programmatic assessment. These development activities should not focus only on information-based sessions but provide hands-on venues for the teachers to actively engage in the development and implementation process.
4. Feedback is the cornerstone of programmatic assessment, and its value should not be underestimated. Despite strong advocacy of the value of feedback in programmatic assessment, quality feedback is still lacking in many programs. It is a difficult skill that needs time to develop and therefore demands special attention.
5. Many implementation reports suggest that learners find programmatic assessment as a way of partnership with their schools where they feel in control of their learning (also known as *learner's agency*). The teacher-student relationship, however, is very critical for this partnership. The less dominant the teacher is, the more likely it is for the programmatic assessment to succeed. Mentoring program has been found useful for building a meaningful teacher-student relationship.
6. This chapter provides a basic understanding of what programmatic assessment is and why it is an effective and useful alternative assessment approach. We have also provided numerous practical tips to help the readers in the design and implementation process. We anticipate that the readers of this chapter will find this information helpful to their educational practices.

## References

1. Etheridge L, Boursicot K. Performance and workplace assessment. In: A Practical Guide for Medical Teachers. 5th ed. Elsevier; 2017. p. 267–73.
2. van der Vleuten CPM. The assessment of professional competence: Developments, research and practical implications. Adv Heal Sci Educ. 1996;1(1):41–67.
3. Heeneman S, de Jong LH, Dawson LJ, Wilkinson TJ, Ryan A, Tait GR, et al. Ottawa 2020 consensus statement for programmatic assessment – 1. Agreement on the principles. Med Teach. 2021;43(10):1139–48.

4. Cobb KA, Brown G, Jaarsma DADC, Hammond RA. The educational impact of assessment: A comparison of DOPS and MCQs. Med Teach. 2013;35(11):e1598–607.
5. Palmer EJ, Devitt PG. Assessment of higher order cognitive skills in undergraduate education: Modified essay or multiple choice questions? Research paper. BMC Med Educ. 2007;7:1–7.
6. McCoubrie P. Improving the fairness of multiple-choice questions: A literature review. Med Teach. 2004;26(8):709–12.
7. Schuwirth LWT, van der Vleuten CPM. Programmatic assessment and Kane's validity perspective. Med Educ. 2012;46(1):38–48.
8. Munoz LQ, O'Byrne C, Pugsley J, Austin Z. Reliability, validity, and generalizability of an objective structured clinical examination (OSCE) for assessment of entry-to-practice in pharmacy. Pharm Educ. 2005;5(1).
9. van der Vleuten CPM, Schuwirth LWT, Driessen EW, Dijkstra J, Tigelaar D, Baartman LKJ, et al. A model for programmatic assessment fit for purpose. Med Teach. 2012 Mar 25;34(3):205–14.
10. Driessen EW, Van Tartwijk J, Govaerts M, Teunissen P, van der Vleuten CPM. The use of programmatic assessment in the clinical workplace: A Maastricht case report. Med Teach. 2012;34(3):226–31.
11. Schuwirth LWT, van der Vleuten CPM. Programmatic assessment: From assessment of learning to assessment for learning. Med Teach. 2011;33(6):478–85.
12. Murre JMJ, Dros J. Replication and analysis of Ebbinghaus' forgetting curve. PLoS One. 2015;10(7):e0120644.
13. Cilliers FJ, Schuwirth LWT, Herman N, Adendorff HJ, van der Vleuten CPM. A model of the pre-assessment learning effects of summative assessment in medical education. Adv Heal Sci Educ. 2012;17(1):39–53.
14. Bing-You R, Hayes V, Varaklis K, Trowbridge R, Kemp H, McKelvy D. Feedback for learners in medical education: what is known? A scoping review. Acad Med. 2017;92(9):1346–54.
15. van der Vleuten CPM, Schuwirth LWT, Driessen EW, Govaerts MJB, Heeneman S. Twelve tips for programmatic assessment. Med Teach. 2015;37(7):641–6.
16. Timmerman AA, Dijkstra J. A practical approach to programmatic assessment design. Adv Heal Sci Educ. 2017;22(5):1169–82.
17. Heeneman S, Oudkerk Pool A, Schuwirth LWT, van der Vleuten CPM, Driessen EW. The impact of programmatic assessment on student learning: Theory versus practice. Med Educ. 2015;49(5):487–98.
18. De Jong LH, Favier RP, Van der Vleuten CPM, Bok HGJ. Students' motivation toward feedback-seeking in the clinical workplace. Med Teach. 2017;39(9):954–8.
19. Torre DM, Schuwirth LWT, Van der Vleuten CPM. Theoretical considerations on programmatic assessment. Med Teach. 2020;42(2):213–20.
20. Kinsella EA. Professional knowledge and the epistemology of reflective practice. Nurs Philos. 2010;11(1):3–14.
21. Bruner J. Actual minds, possible worlds. Harvard University Press; 2020.
22. Vygotsky LS. Mind in society (M. Cole, V. John-Steiner, S. Scribner, & E. Souberman, Eds.). Cambridge, MA: Harvard University Press; 1978.
23. Feuerstein R, Feuerstein RS, Falik LH, Rand Y. The dynamic assessment of cognitive modifiability: The Learning Propensity Assessment Device: Theory, instruments and techniques, Rev. and exp. ed. of The dynamic assessment of retarded performers. ICELP Publications; 2002.
24. Groot F, Jonker G, Rinia M, ten Cate O, Hoff RG. Simulation at the frontier of the zone of proximal development. Acad Med. 2020;95(7):1098–105.
25. Fernández M, Wegerif R, Mercer N, Rojas-Drummond S. Re-conceptualizing "scaffolding" and the zone of proximal development in the context of symmetrical collaborative learning. J Classr Interact. 2015;50(1):54–72.
26. Schut S, Maggio LA, Heeneman S, van Tartwijk J, van der Vleuten C, Driessen E. Where the rubber meets the road — An integrative review of programmatic assessment in health care professions education. Perspect Med Educ. 2020;6–13.

27. ten Cate O, Chen HC, Hoff RG, Peters H, Bok H, van der Schaaf M. Curriculum development for the workplace using Entrustable Professional Activities (EPAs): AMEE Guide No. 99. Med Teach. 2015;37(11):983–1002.
28. ten Cate O, Taylor DR. The recommended description of an entrustable professional activity: AMEE Guide No. 140. Med Teach. 2021;43(10):1106–14.
29. Schiekirka S, Anders S, Raupach T. Assessment of two different types of bias affecting the results of outcome-based evaluation in undergraduate medical education. BMC Med Educ. 2014;14(1):149.
30. Fuller R, Homer M, Pell G. Longitudinal interrelationships of OSCE station level analyses, quality improvement and overall reliability. Med Teach. 2013;35(6):515–7.
31. van der Vleuten C, Heeneman S, Schuwirth LWT. Programmatic Assessment. In: A Practical Guide for Medical Teachers, 5th Edition. 2017:295-303.
32. Ramani S, Krackov SK. Twelve tips for giving feedback effectively in the clinical environment. Med Teach. 2012;34(10):787–91.
33. Iqbal MZ, Könings KD, Al-Eraky MM, van Merriënboer JJG. Entrustable professional activities for small-group facilitation: a validation study using modified Delphi technique. Teach Learn Med. 2021;33(5):536–45.
34. Iqbal MZ, Könings KD, Al-Eraky M, AlSheikh MH, van Merrienboer JJG. Development of an entrustable professional activities (EPAs) framework for small group facilitators through a participatory design approach. Med Educ Online. 2020;25(1):1694309.

## *Reading Material*

## *We recommend the readers to consult the following resources to advance their knowledge on programmatic assessment.*

Driessen, E. W., Van Tartwijk, J., Govaerts, M., Teunissen, P., & Van Der Vleuten, C. P. M. (2012). The use of programmatic assessment in the clinical workplace: A Maastricht case report. *Medical Teacher*, *34*(3), 226–231.

Schuwirth, L. W. T., & van der Vleuten, C. P. M. (2011). Programmatic assessment: From assessment of learning to assessment for learning. *Medical Teacher*, *33*(6), 478–485.

Torre, D. M., Schuwirth, L. W. T., & van der Vleuten, C. P. M. (2020). Theoretical considerations on programmatic assessment. *Medical Teacher*, *42*(2), 213–220.

van der Vleuten, C., Heeneman, S., & Schuwirth, L. W. T. (2021). Programmatic assessment. *A Practical Guide for Medical Teachers,* Elsevier.

van der Vleuten, C. P. M., Schuwirth, L. W. T., Driessen, E. W., Dijkstra, J., Tigelaar, D., Baartman, L. K. J., & Van Tartwijk, J. (2012). A model for programmatic assessment fit for purpose. *Medical Teacher*, *34*(3), 205–214.

van der Vleuten, C. P. M., Schuwirth, L. W. T., Driessen, E. W., Govaerts, M. J. B., & Heeneman, S. (2015). Twelve tips for programmatic assessment. *Medical Teacher*, *37*(7), 641–646.

# Chapter 13
# Assessment: Social Accountability and the Society

**Mohamed Elhassan Abdalla**

**Abstract** This chapter addresses a different aspect of students' assessment, that is, the societal role and function. In addition, this chapter discusses the effect of social factors on the development of student's assessment besides the role of assessment in the promotion of institutions' social accountability and other social constructs.

**Keywords** Social accountability · Assessment · Society

There is a strong belief among educators, students, and other society members that the assessment of students is a function of teachers and faculty members in education institutions and that examinations and their questions are largely related to educational culture in institutions [1]. In another side, it is also known that assessment can be considered and studied as a societal function and aspect [1]. In the Chapter named 'Socio-cultural aspects of assessment' in 'Review of Research in Education', Gipps, C. provided a background for the start of assessment. So, historically, examinations were used for the first time in China to select candidates for jobs (206 BC to 220 AD), and assessment was introduced by Jesuits in schools in the seventeenth century. In the medical profession, qualifying exams were firstly introduced in 1817 in Britain to qualify doctors to be members of the profession. Later, exams become more popular from the 1850s. As the demand from middle-class population to enter universities increased, exams were introduced to regulate that entry. From then onward, examinations became part of the education process all over the world, in higher education and general education as well [2].

From that time assessment is continuously developed based on the different social movements, for example, one of the social aspects that govern the assessment and lead to the development of objective tests such as Multiple-Choice Questions (MCQs) and the Objective Structured Clinical Examination (OSCE) is the concept and the social movement of equity between all individuals in the society

M. E. Abdalla (✉)
School of Medicine, University of Limerick, Limerick, Ireland
e-mail: MElhassan.Elsayed@ul.ie



H. E. E. Gasmalla et al. (eds.), *Written Assessment in Medical Education*,
https://doi.org/10.1007/978-3-031-11752-7_13

[2]. Hence, assessment has effects and changes in society and at the same time society has a role to play in the assessment process. This chapter aims to present the societal aspects of assessment to the reader.

Assessment of students is defined as "the process of generating, gathering, recording, interpreting, using and reporting evidence of learning in individuals, groups or systems. Educational assessment provides information about progress in learning, and achievement in developing skills, knowledge, behaviours and attitudes" [3]. The functions of assessment depend on the type of assessment practiced: assessment of learning or assessment for learning with its subdivision assessment as learning. Assessment of learning refers to the summative assessment that ends with marking and grading, assessment for learning is an assessment that is designed to provide feedback to students about their progress in learning, while assessment as learning is the assessment type that engages student's metacognition [4].

Understanding students' assessment has two sides: understanding from the teachers' point of view and understanding from the society's point of view. Teachers concentrate on fairness, assessment purpose, and how to fit with the grading system within the institution. While society considers the outcome of the assessment in terms of the quality of graduates and the sociocultural aspects of the assessment results, those sociocultural aspects of assessment can shape the assessment policies and practice differently based on geographical and social differences [4]. The social aspects of assessment can set rules for the practice of assessment within the institute [5]. Unfortunately, up-to-date literature on health professions education offers few examples of the effect of society's role on student assessment and the accountability of health professions education to the society through assessment.

In 1995, the World Health Organization has made the definition for social accountability of medical schools [SA] as "the obligation [of medical schools] to direct their education, research and service activities towards addressing the priority health concerns of the community, region, and/or nation they have the mandate to serve" [6]. Although the definition was for medical schools but it can be applied to all health professions education.

The definition of Social Accountability together with the Global Consensus on Social Accountability of Medical Schools (GCSA) that published in 2010 call for reform in curricula to fit with the changing health needs of the societies [7]. The GCSA sets ten strategic directions to move toward social accountability: direction No. 3 calls for adapting to the evolving roles of doctors and other health professionals and direction No. 4 calls for fostering outcome-based education. Application of those two directions needs transformation on the existing curricula and consideration when developing new ones. Obviously, the transformation should take into consideration all aspects of curriculum including assessment. This transformation – when happen – will provide an obvious example of how social issues can affect and influence change in the assessment.

To imply assessment that fits the transformation to social accountability, thinking beyond the single assessment instrument and/or individual learning outcome is needed. Programmatic assessment may be a better option in this case, where instruments may complete each other to optimize assessment with the function of the program [8], which is, responding to the society's health needs by producing efficient and safe doctors. It also needs to consider validity to give a strong meaning to the assessment [9] that addresses social accountability. In this aspect, concentration on construct validity as the main concept of assessment validity is important. In addition to content validity, construct validity is important in health professions education as social science [9]. In theory, construct validity is used to make meaningful inferences from assessment to the domain of population interest [9]. The domain with social accountability will be the characteristic of the graduate who can satisfy the changing society's needs [10]. The assessment in such transformation needs to have a strong link between the assessment scores and the concept of social accountability that determines the shape of the curriculum and hence the characteristics of the graduate [11].

To observe Social Accountability of health professions education institutions, another measurement must be added to the quality of assessment, that is, the measurement of assessment methods and questions against the values of relevance, quality, equity and cost-effectiveness which are the four values of social accountability govern the education, research and service functions of medical/health professions education institutions-: [6]. This needs to change from the ordinary forms of assessment blueprints health professions institutions used to use to new one that accommodates the four values which were set for the content of the curriculum as an educational function of the medical school, but we need to use them to drive assessment also. For example, with relevance, we need to consider how assessment reflects the diversity of society by enquiring priority health concerns first. For equity, we need to consider that questions do not deprive any category of being represented in the exam questions, for example, women.

As the concept of social accountability needs more work to be part of the health professions education culture and practice [12], then assessment as learning needs to be considered when developing the individual questions. For example, in MCQ stems, it is crucial to include the social determinants of health as part of the scenario. The WHO defines social determinants of health as the conditions in which people are born, grow, live, work, and age; those conditions will affect an individual's health outcomes [13].

Including such information in the questions' stem should not be a nonfunctional wording that adds to the reading time but should be an integral part of the question that has a role in determining the right answer. Ozone et al. [14] stated that students do not consider important social determinants of health in reporting about addiction, unemployment, and social gradient in patients [14]. So, it is significant to add learning about the social determinant of health during teaching and learning and in the assessment. In a review published in 2019 [15] about teaching and learning of social determinant of health, it is found that the assessment is mainly self-reported and few studies reported assessment of the learner outcomes in exams, which means social determinant of health is still not well addressed in all assessment types. This ill-representation in assessment may result in reduced uptake of the concept as learning outcomes by students.

The assessment that considers social determinants of health needs to address the demonstration of achievement of competencies related to transformative learning [16]. The definition of transformative learning reported by Doobay-Persaud et al. in

2019 [15] is the theory of learning that is beyond basic knowledge or skill acquisition whereby the learner's assumptions and perspectives are transformed through experiential learning, facilitated structured reflective dialogue, and high-level analysis. These new beliefs and insights are then applied to current and future actions and critically assessed. This somehow complicated definition implies a different way of thinking that needs to be used in inference from different instruments to judge the achievement of the competencies: 360-degree assessment [16].

Another dimension is needed to increase the sensitivity of assessment and all aspects of health professions education is considering diversity to ensure equity to all patients and populations. Discrimination can have a negative impact that leads to health inequality and the access to health services by minorities [17]. The issue of diversity needs to be addressed to promote it as a culture among students [18] and should be reflected both in curriculum content and assessment [19]. There is no standard way for including diversity in assessment [19], but if it is not taken into consideration, assessment can create bias against minority groups [20] or persons with different colors and cultural backgrounds. It is the role of teachers to be conscious of including questions scenarios as well as OSCE stations that reflect a diversity of patients. This consciousness is crucial for the future practice as a study in dermatology assessment in Canada revealed that students are more confident when facing a question with white skin compared to skin of color [21] as a result of the lack of representation of skin of color in the dermatology teaching in North America as stated by authors. Most of the guidelines for question construction recommend including demographic data to make scenarios as real as possible. The challenge now is to make sure that the demographic data will reflect the diversity and social determinants of health.

Besides all the abovementioned considerations, in assessments that consider social accountability or being sensitive to the society, teachers need to consider many aspects related to the society where the instruction is located such as the interpretation wording [20]. This is crucial nowadays specially with the use of the international questions banks shared by different institutions, the use of international assessments, or use of examination from another institution for the purpose of benchmarking.

In conclusion, assessment is meant to measure students' achievement of the planned curriculum learning outcome, but it has more to support social accountability and other social concepts. Teachers needs to think beyond classrooms when developing exam questions.

**Take-Home Message**

Assessment is not only for measuring student's learning outcomes inside the classroom, it has a social role that needs to be considered by teachers and faculty members when planning and designing the questions for examinations.

## References


1. Abulencia AS. The Social Purposes of Learning Assessment. ATIKAN. 2011;1(1).
2. Gipps C. Chapter 10: Socio-cultural aspects of assessment. Rev Res Educ. 1999;24(1):355–92.
3. National Council for Curriculum and Assessment. Glossary [Internet]. 2022 [cited 2022 May 3]. Available from: https://ncca.ie/en/junior-cycle/assessment-and-reporting/glossary/#:~:text=Glossary-,Assessment,%2C knowledge%2C behaviours and attitudes.
4. DeLuca C, Rickey N, Coombs A. Exploring assessment across cultures: Teachers' approaches to assessment in the U.S., China, and Canada. Fai Hui SK, editor. Cogent Educ [Internet]. 2021 Jan 1;8(1). Available from: https://www.tandfonline.com/doi/full/10.1080/2331186X.2021.1921903
5. Xu Y, Brown GTL. Teacher assessment literacy in practice: A reconceptualization. Teach Teach Educ [Internet]. 2016 Aug;58:149–62. Available from: https://linkinghub.elsevier.com/retrieve/pii/S0742051X16300907
6. Boelen C, Heck J. Defining and measuring the social accountability of medical schools [Internet]. Geneva, Switzerland: Division of Development of Human Resources for Health; 1995. Available from: https://apps.who.int/iris/handle/10665/59441
7. GCSA. Global Consensus for Social Accountability of Medical Schools [Internet]. Vol. 2011, Global Consensus for Social Accountability of Medical Schools. 2010 [cited 2018 Oct 2]. Available from: http://healthsocialaccountability.sites.olt.ubc.ca/files/2011/06/11-06-07-GCSA-English-pdf-style.pdf
8. Van Der Vleuten CPM, Schuwirth LWT, Driessen EW, Govaerts MJB, Heeneman S. Twelve Tips for programmatic assessment. Med Teach [Internet]. 2015 Jul 3;37(7):641–6. Available from: http://www.tandfonline.com/doi/full/10.3109/0142159X.2014.973388
9. Downing S. Validity: on the meaningful interpretation of assessment data. Med Educ. 2003;37:830–837.
10. Frenk J, Chen L, Bhutta ZA, Cohen J, Crisp N, Evans T, et al. Health professionals for a new century: transforming education to strengthen health systems in an interdependent world. Lancet. 2010;376(9756):1923–58.
11. Abdalla ME. Suggested new standards to measure social accountability of medical schools in the accreditation systems. J Case Stud Accredit Assess [Internet]. 2014;3. Available from: http://www.aabri.com/manuscripts/131505.pdf
12. Abdalla ME, Boelen C, Osman WN. Development and evaluation of an online course about the social accountability of medical schools. J Taibah Univ Med Sci. 2019;14(3).
13. World Health Organization. Social Determinant of Health [Internet]. [cited 2022 May 5]. Available from: https://www.who.int/health-topics/social-determinants-of-health#tab=tab_1
14. Ozone S, Haruta J, Takayashiki A, Maeno T, Maeno T. Students' understanding of social determinants of health in a community-based curriculum: a general inductive approach for qualitative data analysis. BMC Med Educ [Internet]. 2020;20(1):470. Available from: https://doi.org/10.1186/s12909-020-02391-z
15. Doobay-Persaud A, Adler MD, Bartell TR, Sheneman NE, Martinez MD, Mangold KA, et al. Teaching the Social Determinants of Health in Undergraduate Medical Education: a Scoping Review. J Gen Intern Med [Internet]. 2019 May 16;34(5):720–30. Available from: http://link.springer.com/10.1007/s11606-019-04876-0
16. Social Determinants of Health: A Framework for Educating Health Professionals. In: A Framework for Educating Health Professionals to Address the Social Determinants of Health [Internet]. Washington, D.C.: National Academies Press; 2016. Available from: https://www.nap.edu/catalog/21923
17. Hall WJ, Chapman M V., Lee KM, Merino YM, Thomas TW, Payne BK, et al. Implicit Racial/Ethnic Bias Among Health Care Professionals and Its Influence on Health Care Outcomes: A Systematic Review. Am J Public Health [Internet]. 2015 Dec;105(12):e60–76. Available from: http://ajph.aphapublications.org/doi/10.2105/AJPH.2015.302903

18. Muntinga ME, Krajenbrink VQE, Peerdeman SM, Croiset G, Verdonk P. Toward diversity-responsive medical education: taking an intersectionality-based approach to a curriculum evaluation. Adv Heal Sci Educ [Internet]. 2016 Aug 24;21(3):541–59. Available from: http://link.springer.com/10.1007/s10459-015-9650-9
19. Dutta N, Maini A, Afolabi F, Forrest D, Golding B, Salami RK, et al. Promoting cultural diversity and inclusion in undergraduate primary care education. Educ Prim Care [Internet]. 2021 Jul 4;32(4):192–7. Available from: https://www.tandfonline.com/doi/full/10.1080/14739879.2021.1900749
20. Kim KH, Zabelina D. Cultural bias in assessment: Can creativity assessment help? Int J Crit Pedagog. 2015;6(2).
21. Bellicoso E, Quick SO, Ayoo KO, Beach RA, Joseph M, Dahlke E. Diversity in Dermatology? An Assessment of Undergraduate Medical Education. J Cutan Med Surg [Internet]. 2021 Jul 13;25(4):409–17. Available from: http://journals.sagepub.com/doi/10.1177/12034754211007430

# Index






H. E. E. Gasmalla et al. (eds.), *Written Assessment in Medical Education*, https://doi.org/10.1007/978-3-031-11752-7

The manufacturer's authorised representative in the EU is Springer Nature Customer Service Centre GmbH, Europaplatz 3, 69115 Heidelberg, Germany. If you have any concerns regarding our products, please contact ProductSafety@springernature.com

Printed and bound by CPI Group (UK) Ltd, Croydon, CR0 4YY
01/10/2026
02225893-0019